Praise for
Suffering to Thriving

I was told my breast cancer had returned as metastatic stage 4 cancer and that I was terminal. A year later my doctor was surprised by how clear the scan results looked. The only treatment I used was based on Kathy's wisdom, experience, and inspiration.

Her words gave me the knowledge, hope, and determination that helped me heal myself. All of the healing treatments she brings out in her book *do* work.

She helped me fight cancer and continue living to the fullest.
—Kristy Frazier

Kathy is able to use her pain to help others navigate their issues by showing them how to be their own medical advocate. Being able to witness this in a small part has been nothing short of inspiring and encouraging.
—Dr. Kenneth C. Browning, DO

Your tips and toolbox are gold. Every human being will find value in this book.
—Maia Bell

I love your book! I found out things I didn't know. Your book will change many people's lives.
—Beverly Johnson, RN, PsyD

I am so grateful I have Kathy (and her book) in my life to remind me to trust my intuition about my health. Before getting my lupus diagnosis, I was so frustrated with my body and mental health. Through Kathy's guidance on how to prepare for my medical appointments and what questions to ask, I've already begun seeing huge improvements in my health in only two months. Thank you!
—Kim Negrete

Kathy's strategies for managing severe pain got me through countless hours of agony in the first few weeks of a long recovery from severe injury. When the meds just weren't strong enough, I had Kathy's tools to help me quell the panic that only magnified the pain. Her hard-won wisdom got me through many desperate hours. I am beyond grateful.

—Carolyn Stevens

Living with chronic pain is a complex and isolating experience. Kathy's insights are not only practical but have provided the framework I need to create a path of productivity and hope.

—Danielle Segura

I am blessed to call Kathy a friend, mentor, and soul sister. Her guidance through my healing journey has been invaluable. She has a wealth of firsthand knowledge about the trials and tribulations of this process, and she shares her wisdom openly. She will accompany you on your path to hope and healing. What a treasure to have everything compiled in this book.

—Brandy Dyess

I was amazed how this book hit home on so many different levels. I'm a caretaker for older parents and the support team for my best friends and all the crises they have. Instead of putting myself first, I always put myself last. I go throughout the day with my paper plate smile on the outside but on the inside, I'm hiding my mental, physical, and emotional pain. This book has helped me discover that I need to take time for myself and help myself as much as I help others.

—Teresa Johnson

After close to a year of only being able to walk in excruciating pain, I found that Kathy's empathy, wisdom, and advice helped me reach a decision that led me on the path toward recovery. I am incredibly grateful.

—Kirsten Stewart

When I think of Kathy's book and wisdom, I think of compassion, wisdom, and belief. She embodies the compassion to want to help others feel better and heal, the wisdom to put together a book that shares and guides us on our journey of healing, and the belief that we can do this. We can get through our suffering and enjoy life with Kathy as our guide.

—Wendy Ruth

In her tender connection with the universe, Kathy shares with us her dedication and exploration of a remarkable journey of healing. Pure and authentic. We, as she, become our own healers.

—C. O'Neil

Suffering to Thriving

Your Toolkit for Navigating Your Healing Journey

How to Live a More Healthy, Peaceful, Joyful Life

Kathy Harmon-Luber

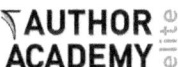

Suffering to Thriving: Your Toolkit for Navigating Your Healing Journey © 2022 by Kathy Harmon-Luber.
All rights reserved.

Published by Author Academy Elite
PO Box 43, Powell, OH 43065
www.AuthorAcademyElite.com

All rights reserved. This book contains material protected under international and federal copyright laws and treaties. Any unauthorized reprint or use of this material is prohibited. No part of this book may be reproduced or transmitted in any form or by any means, electronic or mechanical, including photocopying, recording, or by any information storage and retrieval system, without express written permission from the author.

This book is intended as an informational guide and is not meant to diagnose, treat, or prescribe any condition or replace any medical advice or treatments. Always consult your physician and/or other health care providers. Neither the author nor publisher accepts any responsibility for how you choose to use the information contained herein.

Identifiers:
LCCN: 2022902601
ISBN: 979-8-88583-015-7 (paperback)
ISBN: 979-8-88583-016-4 (hardback)
ISBN: 979-8-88583-017-1 (ebook)

Available in paperback, hardback, e-book, and audiobook

Any Internet addresses (websites, blogs, etc.) and telephone numbers printed in this book are offered as a resource. They are not intended in any way to be or imply an endorsement by Author Academy Elite, nor does Author Academy Elite vouch for the content of these sites and numbers for the life of this book.

Dedication

To Ken, who has walked every step of this journey by my side with his heart full of love and patience.

To Carolyn and Joyce for creating the Healing Journey Fellowship, and to Heléne and other Fellowship[1] supporters who made this book possible.

To friends and family, thank you for your love, compassion, and enthusiastic support.

To the medical professionals, especially Dr. Kenneth C. Browning, DO, and lifestyle coach Jodi Sutherland.

To everyone on the healing journey who dreams of a better life. May this book be a roadmap to healing.

To Mother Earth and our Creator for our abundant blessings.

Quiet friend who has come so far,

feel how your breathing makes more space around you.
Let this darkness be a belltower
and you the bell. As you ring,

what batters you becomes your strength.

—Rainer Maria Rilke,
"Let this Darkness Be a Belltower"

TABLE OF CONTENTS

Introduction xv

PART 1:
UNDERSTANDING SUFFERING

1 Everybody Hurts 3

2 This Thing Called Suffering. 7

PART 2:
THE THRIVING MINDSET

3 This Too Shall Pass 15

4 Make Your Mind Your Medicine 19

5 Which Wolf Are You Feeding?. 25

6 In This Moment 29

7 Change Your Mind. 35

PART 3:
PREPARING YOUR MIND AND SPIRIT

8 There Will Be Tears. 47

9	A Stampede of Horses: Pain	53
10	Surviving Isolation: Housebound Shut-in to Lit-up Homebody	67
11	Yes, Please!	75

PART 4:
YOUR SELF-DIRECTED HEALING JOURNEY

12	Compass Intuition: Learning to Listen	81
13	Fight for It: Robust Self-Care	93
14	Taking Inventory: Ability, not Disability	99
15	Maximize Your Medical Appointment	107
16	Super Sleuthy You	115
17	Stick-With-It-Ness	127
18	Bears Do It, Bees Do It	131

PART 5:
THE THRIVING SPIRIT

19	Keys to Peace: Acceptance, Surrender, and Letting Go	141
20	Surrounded by Sharks: Holding onto Hope	153
21	Courageously Dare to Heal	157
22	Ever Always Gratitude	161
23	Fear vs. Love	167
24	Wonder-Filled	171

25 RX: Laughter 175

26 Sparkling Resilience 177

PART 6:
THE THRIVING TOOLKIT

27 Transformation: Sitting in Darkness Like a Caterpillar 187

28 Write a Different Ending 193

29 Monk Morning. 199

30 Healing Power of Art 203

31 Practicing Peace 209

32 Talking to Myself: Intentions 215

33 Inner Sanctuary 217

34 You Wild Thing 221

35 Day Tripping: Don't Give Up Your Dreams 229

36 The Guided Journey: Visualization & Meditation . . . 235

37 Good Vibrations. 247

38 Bon Voyage 253

Acknowledgments. 255

About the Author 257

Next Steps on Your Healing Journey 259

Endnotes 261

INTRODUCTION

> Although the world is full of suffering,
> it is full also of the overcoming of it.
>
> —Helen Keller

Standing in our kitchen, waiting for the coffee to brew, I was chatting with my husband when searing pain, like an electrical shock, bolted through my lower back. It took my breath away.

In that one moment, my entire life changed drastically—never to be the same. Blinded by tears, barely able to stand on my own, I shakily hobbled to our bedroom to lie down. It was 9:10 a.m. on December 8, 2016.

I immediately recognized this pain as a spinal disc rupture (the bursting of the shock-absorbing jelly donut between two vertebrae). In my case, this disc jelly—which causes inflammation to the spinal cord and surrounding tissue—glommed onto the sciatic nerve running down my left leg. Thus the debilitating pain.

I had a routine checkup with my GP already scheduled for later that day. By that afternoon, however, I was unable to get out of bed. Not that day. Not the next day. Not for months.

Here is an excerpt from one of my journal entries:

December 8, 2016—my year-end buzz-kill disc rupture journey of lessons. *I have always loved the shape of the crescent moon. Now, it's the most comfortable position of my body, lying in bed so my back and left leg are not in screaming pain . . . head and feet to my right side, hips pushed out to my left. It takes the pressure off of the disc. However romantic that crescent moon image is, I'm writhing in pain. I've had these disc ruptures before . . . never this level of pain. Off the charts. Agony.*

It was the fourth disc rupture I had suffered in two decades, complicated and made inoperable by several hereditary spinal diseases—diagnosed decades ago, in my twenties—converging in a perfect storm.

That was five years ago, and now as I write this book, I am lying on the same bed, supported by a system of orthopedic pillows. I've made great progress, and I'm happy to say that today I'm thriving.

Ever the optimist, back then I was certain I'd be all better a few days after the rupture. But a week later, I painfully struggled to get out of bed and walk nine steps to the master bathroom. I couldn't make it to the bedroom door, let alone get to the doctor's office. Day and night I was flat on my back, but at the two-week mark, I was sure I'd be up and back to normal in a month.

Day 31. Day 32 . . . Day 365, and I was still laid out flat. When I was finally physically able to get to an appointment with a top neurosurgeon, he—like the seven orthopedic surgeons before him—wouldn't operate. I was told it would be a fourteen-plus-hour surgery to "rebuild" my back with shitty risky odds: 40 percent chance I'd have less pain and more mobility, high risk of paralysis. *No thank you.*

When I asked, "Now what?" he said the new thinking is, "If it's healing at all on its own, no surgery." He advised rest . . . anywhere from six months to three years.

I cheerily responded, "I'm an overachiever; I'll be fine in six months." I wasn't.

When I was twenty-one, orthopedic doctors told me that by my mid-thirties I'd be in a wheelchair. Now, lying there in bed day in, day out, doubt began seeping into my brain: *Has it finally happened? Will I be bedridden for the rest of my life? Wheelchair-bound?*

Horribly destabilizing and debilitating, the rupture left me bedridden and in devastating pain for five years . . . and counting. Thankfully, I have avoided the wheelchair. What's most amazing is that I managed to work during this whole period of recovery, anywhere from twenty to fifty or more hours a week. You guessed it: all from bed because immobilization is a vital part of my daily pain management. It's also the consolation prize for not living life from a wheelchair.

Finding the Road to Thriving

Up until the instant of the rupture, I had been very active: hiking in the mountains we call home, traveling abroad, swimming, dancing, and spending time in nature. I was a writer for nonprofit organizations making a difference in the world, an award-winning fine-art photographer, a painter, a professional classical flute musician and teacher, a board member of community organizations, a wife, a daughter, a stepmom, a sister, and a friend.

I went from living the life of my dreams to a life that felt small—a health crisis and a life catastrophe followed by isolation and suffering. As an active person who's had her share of sports and dance injuries, I thought I knew pain, but I'd never known anything as agonizing as this.

I was afraid.

You can probably relate to the pain, suffering, loss, disappointment, and depression brought on by illness, injury, or chronic disease. Deep suffering, both physical and mental, moved in and put down roots. Initially, I was so overwhelmed I lost touch with what I already knew about the healing path. Then, slowly, I began to reclaim my knowledge of healing. For a time, I vacillated on and off the path I knew led to well-being, but the way out of suffering began gradually to appear, carved out of the darkness in the mist of tears, despair, and self-pity. I became more successful at choosing to be on the path of healing.

The good news is, even while bedridden, I discovered how to get from suffering to thriving, and now I live a more peaceful, joyful, and hope-filled life. And you can too.

I won't sugarcoat it: I was miserable, in the pit of despair. The way to thriving was anything but easy. But now I *know* the way—and I'm eager to share it with you.

Health crises break the rhythm of our lives, but they can be a portal to a better life full of new opportunities. I wrote a different ending to my story. That's what this book is about . . . walking through the gateway of your health crisis and finding a better story for your life. I'll show you how to embrace your healing journey and find a new way of being in the world: more hope, more joy, more peace. It's a road map for how to love your life.

My healing journey began in earnest in my thirties. That's when I learned I could heal myself from many things: asthma, chronic sinus infections, chronic bronchitis, Raynaud's disease (a progressively worsening, incurable autoimmune disease), allergies, torn menisci in my knees, chronic depression and anxiety disorder, kidney stones, and arthritis. This was when I got into vibrational medicine, which I was intrigued to find had both traditional and scientific backing. I learned our thoughts are vibrations that can change our lives; while the body is suffering, the mind need not.

To be clear, Western medicine has saved my life on numerous occasions. However, this is a story of how complementary medicine (or natural healing protocols, many of which are thousands of years old) used *along with* Western protocols healed me, built up my immunity, and prevented disease progression.

I'm no doctor, but I do know this much is true: the body's healing presents an opportunity to heal your soul. This is a healing journey within a life journey within your soul's journey. Coping with a health crisis can be transformational spiritually (whatever your spiritual belief is—or isn't). It's possible to transcend suffering and thrive.

Face it, we don't know what we don't know. And when we're suffering, it's like the Buddhist adage—we're "looking at the sky through a straw." There's so much we don't see. It's a narrow view of what's out there, what's possible.

So when someone comes along and points to something you didn't see—or takes away the straw you've been looking through—it can be a great gift, often transformational. When I started on this path, I learned self-discovery aids the healing journey. There was *so* much I didn't know. When others recommended some treatment, pointed out an issue I wasn't aware of, or suggested a way of shifting perspective on a problem, I researched, investigated, experimented, and tracked my progress. I soon began walking a new path. Over time, glimmers of light, peace, hope, and joy grew, giving me the courage to continue. We're far more resilient than we realize. We can build resilience like a muscle.

Walking the healing path has become my life's purpose, and now, I've got the bird's-eye view. I'll share this to help you rise above your suffering to find the aerial perspective—a better view of your own healing journey and life purpose.

What This Book Is About

Is your suffering (pain, illness, injury, disease, loss, or even old age) holding you back from living your best life? Health crises—whether physical, emotional, or spiritual—are territories for which we have no map. We didn't receive one at birth or when we graduated high school. This book is a guide to help you navigate the often difficult, challenging healing journey—a Toolkit to help you maximize your healing potential. Pick the right tool for what you need when you need it. Use this time to ask deeper questions and build a new life with new tools. It's the book I wish I had decades ago.

This book will help you learn to:

- Embrace your health crisis as a teacher on your life's journey and soul's journey.
- Understand how your healing journey aligns with your life's journey and your soul's journey.
- Emerge from the darkness of pain, loss, disappointment, despair, and depression.
- Discover new wisdom, insights, strengths, passions, and purpose.
- Find a path out of suffering not to merely survive but thrive.
- Achieve more peace and happiness.
- See the silver lining and write a new story for your future.
- Take setbacks in stride with better resilience.
- Find acceptance—gratitude even—for the experience.

I hope this book will serve as a map of the rough terrain so you don't get lost in it, a trail of breadcrumbs strategically placed so you can find your way through it, and a navigation system to help you heal and cope when you're stuck. I'll show you how.

I'm meeting you where you are on your healing journey. Whether you're at the first step of getting a diagnosis or have been struggling for years, you'll benefit. To change our future, we need to change our mind, build our own map, try a new road, and use our own compass. The information you find here might offer a new way of thinking. Or perhaps it will be a reminder of what you already know. Be open. Be ready to try something different.

As Albert Einstein once said (I'm paraphrasing here), if we want a different result, we need to try a new way of doing things. Take my hand—wander through this book with me.

How to Use This Book

You'll find six parts:

- **Part 1: Understanding Suffering.** Illness and injury are facts of life. At some point, they happen to everyone—young, middle-aged, or elderly. In this section, we'll look at the human condition and how suffering is a natural reaction to pain, be it physical or mental. We'll get out of the weeds of daily suffering by taking an aerial view of our health crisis as a pathway to more robust, transformational personal development.

- **Part 2: The Thriving Mindset.** Chapters on the stages of healing will provide practical guidance on how to transcend suffering and develop new beliefs to help healing begin.

- **Part 3: Preparing Your Mind and Spirit.** We'll delve into the challenges of healing in our culture and learn practical things we can do when reality isn't what we wanted it to be.

- **Part 4: Your Self-Directed Healing Journey.** I present my guiding principles of healing and explain how to construct your own healing journey.

- **Part 5: The Thriving Spirit.** I'll teach you how to cultivate and nurture the virtues vital to thriving no matter your circumstances.

- **Part 6: The Thriving Toolkit.** Here I'll present holistic, transformative practices that can help you build resilience and well-being. Here's where you get to play super sleuth and try on what might fit into your healing journey and help you live a more peaceful, joyful, hope-filled life.

Don't feel you must read sequentially, cover-to-cover, as you would most books (although you certainly can do that). If you're short on time and have an immediate need, find a chapter that speaks to you and dive right in. Be certain to review the Table of Contents as some topics covered in earlier chapters have a deeper dive later on.

Throughout this book, I invite you to ponder key questions or to complete small exercises. I believe all progress—in work, play, learning, and health—is incremental. Even micro-practices can yield big gains. Martha Beck describes this process as "one-degree turns toward doing what I really wanted."[2] This book will help you take one-degree turns in your quest for better health. These questions and exercises are easy to contemplate upon waking or before bedtime, while cooking or cleaning, in the shower, or on your walk. If you're bedridden, weave them into your day as an uplifting respite. Allow them to fit into your day organically.

See what small practices resonate with you and build them into your daily practice. Commit to this, and you'll find the changes to be transformative.

Wouldn't you give your best friend, partner, or child the time and energy to help them not only heal but thrive? You are precious. Gift yourself the time and tools to heal. As they tell us in the airplane about those oxygen masks, *take care of yourself first so you can be there for others.*

There are no right or wrong answers to the exercises in this book. They're about excavating your authentic self and Inner Healer and finding what works for you. Take it at your own pace. Dig deep. Sift through the debris you discover. Don't stress about it. That kind of stress just makes healing harder.

The key is to experiment, play, and be curious. I've been doing these practices for decades, and they've changed my health and life for the better. In the beginning, I found it super helpful to keep a journal logging the date, what I tried, observations on what worked and what didn't, wisdom that came to me, and new ideas to explore. Even if you're not a "journal person," give it a try as you begin to work with the tools.

Now, a word about what this book is not: it's not another long to-do list, a book of "shoulds," or formulas to memorize. It's not a religious book (although a handful of quotes have a Buddhist flavor, it doesn't espouse any particular belief system).

Rather, it's a collection of tools I've curated and tested through lived experience. It's more than just my story; it's written for you, with compassion and love, from a place of vulnerability and courage as I hold space for you to heal.

You're not alone in your pain. Millions have walked this path before us and found peace and healing. Believe that you can too.

If this book gives you or a loved one hope, assists your healing, or helps transform your life, then I will have achieved my purpose. It's like the starfish story: a woman walked along a beach where hundreds of starfish had washed up. She followed the surf line, periodically picking up a starfish and tossing it back into the sea. A young man asked her, "Why are you doing this? It's futile. There are hundreds of them; you won't make a difference." As she tossed another back, she replied, "It made a difference to *that* one."

This book is for you, my starfish.

The Road to Thriving

> Be patient where you sit in the dark. Dawn is coming.
> —Rumi

It's easy to get lost in suffering, but there's no need to *stay* lost in suffering. You deserve something better. Are you ready to try something new? Are you ready to dial in your resilience? Are you ready to believe you have a greater life purpose? Then it's time to seek a new path.

I'm not a medical professional but rather someone—like you—who wants to heal, thrive, and live a full and happy life. In these years of convalescence, I have studied and learned many healing modalities: from ancient therapeutic wisdom in cultures all over the world to modern medical advances.

What I offer you are the gifts and enlightenment of my search that helped me lift my spirit to a healing peace, warm my heart with light and gratitude, and fill my body with the need to press forward with an unconditional, some would say mystical, will to sanctify life.

So take my hand. Let's get the heck out of *suffering* and set out toward your next destination: *thriving*. I know this path well. The trailhead is right over there on the next page. Let's go.

PART 1

Understanding Suffering

If we are facing in the right direction,
all we have to do is keep walking.

—Buddhist proverb

1

EVERYBODY HURTS

> Everybody hurts sometimes . . .
> If you feel like you're alone
> No, no, no, you are not alone.
>
> —R.E.M., "Everybody Hurts"

When we're young, we feel invincible. We peer into our future imagining we'll always be twenty-four, strong, independent, and active. But as we mature, we come to recognize that *everything changes*. This was the hard lesson we all had to confront in 2020 with the COVID-19 pandemic and, in the US, the summer of racially charged events. We'll be living with the terrible toll of that year for a long time: the prolonged social isolation, loss of loved ones, economic distress, job loss and financial insecurity, racial inequity, wildfires, hurricanes and other climate change events, political polarity, etc. The challenge for us all is to learn that *everything changes. We are not invincible. Everybody hurts.*

Our vulnerable bodies can be as fragile as glass. Life isn't always fair. Illness and injury are as much a part of life as birth, death, and taxes. Everybody hurts, yes, but it's also true that everybody heals. Everybody will take a healing journey in their lives.

Still, when our own health changes, we're shocked. *How could this happen to me?!* It feels like the end of the world as we know it. Sometimes it is. Everything feels radically different and completely out of our control.

You are not alone, though it can often feel that way. According to the Centers for Disease Control and Prevention, six in ten American adults have a chronic disease.[3] How many more experience a medical crisis on any given day? It's only our culture that makes us feel alone. As prevalent as health crises are, our society tends to ignore the seriously ill, injured, elderly, disabled, and dying. We treat suffering as weakness, and we learn from a young age to fear illness and injury, to hide it, to medicate it.

Society, employers, advertising, and sometimes our own families often wish to airbrush the healing journey—and those of us on it—out of the otherwise "perfect" picture. Everything is supposed to be "fine," right? Meanwhile, we become invisible, exiled by our illness. Left out as the world carries on, suffering alone in silence.

Then there are those who, perhaps unable to deal with their own discomfort and vulnerability, mock and bully, shame or judge. We may feel like misfits who don't belong, deficient in some way.

Here's the real human truth: the healing journey is a rite of passage and an initiation. It's the human condition. Every person alive is on a healing journey of some degree of severity. Illness doesn't discriminate. Young or old, pretty or plain, rich or poor, athlete or couch potato, soul on fire or bored with life . . . eventually, everybody hurts.

Find comfort in the fact that, no matter how you feel in this moment, you are not alone. Remember this.

On the one hand, we're lucky to live in this age of modern medicine. On the other hand, the modern world is taking a harsh toll on our planet—our life support system—and our health. Toxins lurk in our water, air, clothes, and cosmetics, and pesticides hide in our food. The Natural Resources Defense Council reports, "of the more than 80,000 chemicals currently used in the United States, most haven't been adequately tested for their effects on human health."[4] At the same time, toxic stress is everywhere: our jobs, perpetual busyness and overstimulation, the cell phones we cling to, and unending bad news. Combined, these wreak havoc on our health and well-being. No wonder we succumb to disease.

WE TAKE OUR HEALTH FOR GRANTED

I don't know about you, but I grew up believing I'd always be healthy. I took it all for granted. My grandfather, Pop, used to say, "If you have your health, honey, you have everything," but I couldn't comprehend those words back then. I was young, healthy, and active with dance, aerobics, power walking, the gym, biking, swimming, yoga, and a full social-butterfly calendar. I took for granted the simple ability to walk, to play my flute for hours and perform in public, to stand at my artist's easel and paint all day, and to travel with camera in hand. I didn't think about how easily I performed everyday tasks like taking a shower, cooking a meal, putting on a pair of pants, going to lunch with my gal pals, or walking up the stairs to my job.

With my first spinal disc rupture twenty years ago, I learned rather quickly the wisdom of Pop's adage. Without your health, you cannot work, play, be there for your family—or even make a family. Without health, you cannot grow in the direction of your dreams . . . or can you?

EXERCISE

What part of your health or abilities do you take for granted?

For everything you're able to do today, there will come a point when you do it for the last time. That's the reality of life, our fragile bodies, the aging process, and death. Remembering this truth, begin to do things more mindfully. Appreciate what you do have and can do. Start anywhere and build from there. Over time, you'll begin to feel more alive as a result of savoring every moment—all the way until your last.

An easy way to stop taking things, people, or circumstances for granted is to practice negative visualization.[5] Choose something important in your life and then imagine—only for a moment—how your life would change if you didn't have that person or object. Imagine how the loss would impact your health or finances. The point is not to dwell on negative thoughts or to become paranoid but to gain perspective. When you imagine how much worse your life could be, it's hard to continue taking things for granted.

Ironically, negative visualization is an easy way to maintain a positive outlook no matter what happens. (Just don't live in that negative place too long!)

You're completely entitled if you feel that things suck plenty just as they are. But instead of dwelling in those feelings, this exercise allows you to find peace in your situation.

> Change is inevitable, growth is optional.
> —John Maxwell

2
THIS THING CALLED SUFFERING

> We can make ourselves miserable, or we can make ourselves strong. The amount of effort is the same.
>
> —Pema Chödrön

A health crisis or catastrophic injury usually strikes out of left field. Unanticipated. Unwelcome. You're fine one day, and the next, you're thrown off course. Depending on how disastrous it is, it can totally derail your life and leave chaos—or abrupt endings—in its wake.

Most of us feel sorely unprepared for the profound mental and physical suffering and the pain, disappointment, discouragement, and despair that come from health crises. Change is hard. Loss and grief harder still. We likely don't tell ourselves these struggles hold meaning—but they do. Even the downward spiral, rock bottom, or dark night of the soul happens for a reason. Often it's a wake-up call, an initiation.

It's all too easy to get stuck in the mental suffering that overshadows illness and injury. We are snared by what I call "suffering traps." Here are a few of them:

- **Expectation of specific outcomes**—When we expect to be healed in a certain number of days or months, to be able to return to normal life, or to make a complete recovery, we're setting ourselves up to suffer. All that matters is what you can achieve right now—in this moment. Once you accept this, suffering lifts like a weight off your shoulders and soul. And with this inner peace, healing happens.

- **Comparison**—Comparing your Bad Day (of pain, loss, illness, etc.) to someone else's Best Day (similarly, comparing your current inability to your former ability) can cause great suffering. You are not and may never be who you were. And that's okay. You'll find peace when you embrace this.

- **Struggling**—If we don't accept the reality of our situation but instead struggle against it, we'll suffer. You'll endure less pain by living your life with an acceptance of *what is*.

- **Fears and worries**—We suffer less when we face what frightens us. Fears and worries are not truths.

- **Unattainable desire**—On the healing journey, we often desire that our life could be different, and this is often unrealistic. It's certainly not your current reality. When we let go of unattainable desires, suffering evaporates.

- **Allowing "shoulds" to rule**—Illness/injury is your permission slip to walk away from everything you "should do" that no longer serves you (in a responsible way, of course). Make "want-tos" your priority.

- **Perfection**—Holding on to the illusion that your body and health must be perfect creates suffering. As Leonard Cohen sang, "There is a crack, a crack in everything / that's how the light gets in."[6] That crack is imperfection—where light comes into darkness and transforms you. On the darkest moonless night, the stars shine their brightest.

> The sky is filled with stars, invisible by day.
> —Henry Wadsworth Longfellow

Most Suffering Is a Choice

The statement that suffering is a choice may sound insensitive or delusional. We didn't ask for our health crisis; we certainly didn't choose it. But we're talking here about how we respond to things we cannot control. When we let our suffering dominate us, we're putting on what William Blake called "mind-forged manacles."[7]

Suffering can become a prison of our own making wherein we insidiously trap ourselves. We don't need to dwell in that place. Suffering is a choice. The door of the prison of self-imposed suffering is locked from the inside—and you have the key. In other words, it's totally within your power to diminish unnecessary suffering by changing how you perceive and react to it.

Where we place our awareness shapes our reality. If we focus on suffering, our lives become a daily slog through a wasteland of suffering.

In his book *The Stoic Challenge*, William Irvine tells us the goal is "not to remain calm while suffering a setback but rather to experience a setback without thereby suffering."[8] Notice that subtle distinction: suffering and setbacks are not the same thing. We cannot control our health setbacks, but we can control our reactions to them. The body may be in pain, but the mind doesn't need to be. We can be suffering physically yet still be happy to be alive and celebrate beauty, love, friendship, and freedom.

In other words, we live in two worlds—an inner and an outer world, which have significant independence from one another. In the outer world, our bodies may be disabled, diseased, or dying while at the same time our inner world can be lush, vibrant, imaginative, and thriving. Too often people allow terrible challenges in their outer world to overrule their inner world. This is the prison of suffering. We must choose to free ourselves from it. The healing journey can be the catalyst to shift from outer work to inner work.

> Suffering is part of our training program for becoming wise.
> —Ram Dass

Benefits to Suffering?

> Don't turn away. Keep looking at the bandaged place.
> That's where the light enters you.
> —Rumi

It's important that we not turn our eyes from suffering. It may sound strange, I know. But suffering can be a catalyst for change and portal to find:

- greater self-love
- compassion for others who are suffering
- personal growth and development
- spiritual renewal
- resilience

As we'll see in the next chapter, the benefits we gain from the catalyst of suffering can alter the trajectory of our healing.

There's a popular bit of wisdom that says, "Grow through what you go through." On the healing journey, when times are difficult and challenges seem insurmountable, there's always an opportunity to grow. These tests of strength and resilience can be catalysts for finding meaning and purpose in the suffering we go through. Otherwise, what we don't grow through, we learn the hard way through emotional suffering and pain.

There is something sleeping inside you that your health crisis and suffering will awaken—if you let it. You see, your inner world can lie dormant for years—for some people, most of their lives. Sadly, some folks never awaken to their inner world. It usually remains asleep until an event—illness, injury, loss, trauma, or tragedy—awakens it.

Your ailment is the trumpet sounding reveille. Wake up and pay attention!

Some folks are able to transcend their suffering to live a life of meaning and contentment while others become angry, negative, bratty, unkind, and bitter. To become someone who breaks free from this self-imposed prison and thrives, we must aim to cultivate a peaceful, joy-filled, healing inner world. It's a choice. In every moment, we can choose our thoughts and reactions to the ever-present challenges facing us in our exterior world. Choice is the key. To grow and thrive we must choose to end our suffering.

Isn't there enough suffering in the world? If you knew you could get off the path of suffering, wouldn't you? Don't choose to take the suffering road. If you find yourself on it, choose a different way. It's in our power to release ourselves from suffering. We can choose fear or love, craziness or peace, anger or joy, suffering or thriving.

Exercise

I know all this "choice talk" can be hard to swallow. Not too long ago, when people would suggest I had a choice in a given situation, I'd argue with them. "I absolutely did *not* have any choice," I'd say, "I have too much work to do, too many people counting on me, not enough hours in the day . . ." yada, yada.

That was a false belief. Yes, some things happen independent of my volition, but nonetheless, in every moment, I do indeed have *some* choice.

You might be angry, impatient, or in despair because of your condition, and I understand. You're entitled to your feelings; I'm not at all suggesting you ignore or suppress them. Changing your mind means not allowing runaway unproductive thoughts to ruin your health.

You have the power to choose differently, and the following exercise can help you learn what took me many years to discover.

Practice this exercise as often as you need to.

1. **Acknowledge** your health challenges are inviting you to develop a vibrant inner world free of suffering.

2. **Explore** the landscape of your inner world. What are you choosing to suffer through? What is the root of your suffering?

3. **Decide** now that, although you have an illness, you choose to suffer no longer.

4. **Set** your intention today to break free from suffering and enjoy your life.

You'll find more opportunities to work through this process in the chapters ahead.

PART 2

THE THRIVING MINDSET

Nothing goes away until it has taught us what we need to know.

—Pema Chödrön

3
THIS TOO SHALL PASS

Keep some room in your heart for the unimaginable.

—Mary Oliver

In one second, your entire life can change. Reading that, your first thought is probably about a worst-case scenario (especially if you or someone dear to you is seriously ill or has died). But of course, the converse is just as true: in one second our lives can change in the most remarkable, fabulously positive, sweet ways. To think otherwise brings only suffering.

There's a reason we say "this too shall pass" and not simply "this shall pass." The *too* implies the wisdom of experience. We know the territory of pain and injury. And, as the last time, we'll pass through it just fine. Maybe we'll have some new bumps and bruises, but we'll be okay.

I don't know about you, but I find that comforting.

Sometimes we do everything right to take care of ourselves and yet we're miserable. Sometimes what we need is someone to simply listen, hold space for us, and say, "This too shall pass." It's a reminder that tomorrow will be better, and no doubt we'll be wiser, stronger, and more resilient. The sun is always shining behind the clouds.

Nowhere is this more helpful to remember than in the dark night of the soul, which can be brought on by a serious diagnosis, disastrous injury, or painful loss. When I was struggling to cope at one point, I wrote "This too shall pass" on a Post-It note and stuck it to my bathroom mirror. It got me through days, weeks, and months of writhing pain, setback after setback, and medication that made me very sick. It helped me remember it wouldn't always be like this. In the wake of that dark time, I saw a new path, a new way forward, a new calling leading to a new life. This is a transformative soul journey—the caterpillar in the chrysalis . . . alchemy turning silver into gold.

> Well, I must endure the presence of a few caterpillars
> if I wish to become acquainted with the butterflies.
> —Antoine de Saint-Exupery

A horrible moment is often just that—a transitory moment—and illness and pain often ebb and flow. "This too shall pass" underscores the importance of maintaining the aerial view of our lives and not catastrophizing in a bad moment.

What I initially viewed as a setback, I came to accept as a holding pattern, an initiation, essentially a training ground for the rest of my healing journey. While it feels interminable, the holding pattern always passes, and if we do the inner work, we can transcend our situation to arrive at something better.

When we adopt the attitude of *this too shall pass*, we recognize that we're on a roller coaster of emotions and that plummeting to the depths—fear, disappointment, despair, overwhelm, anger, anxiety, grief—will be followed by a more stable plateau, if not rising to new heights. You've overcome setbacks before. You've got this.

The key is patience to endure a lengthy health challenge without giving up. Patience to wait out the storm of setbacks and uncertainty until it passes. Use this time to ask deeper questions and build a new life with new tools.

Exercise

When I tell myself, "This too shall pass," I hear my grandmother Lizzy's comforting voice. Here's something you can do right now in preparation for difficult times: decide whose voice would bring you most reassurance—a family member (alive or not)? a friend? your spouse? your own strong voice? Hear them say

This too shall pass . . .
and tomorrow,
something better!

4

MAKE YOUR MIND YOUR MEDICINE

The universe is change; our life is what our thoughts make it.

—Marcus Aurelius

A barrage of pharmaceutical ads could lead us to believe pills are the only way to heal. Don't get me wrong, meds have saved my life and relieved my pain, but they're not the only way. Plants are medicine. Nature is medicine. And your mind is the most powerful medicine in your Toolkit.

You've probably heard of the mind–body connection. Well, this is the mind-world connection. Our bodies are not separate from our world, after all. In spiritual terms, this is called *manifestation*, the idea that we can change reality with our thoughts.[9] In 2020, manifestation became one of the hottest health and wellness trends. While it actually has roots in the ancient past, today scientists tell us that how we focus our attention rewires our brains.

Healing begins with the right mindset. Your mind informs your body. In other words, your thoughts and emotions influence your body's health. You can manifest better health outcomes with your thoughts.[10]

Your Superpower

> Whether you think you can or you
> think you can't, you're right!
> —Henry Ford

Unfortunately, humans are hardwired to look at what's wrong. According to Michael Singer, "Consciousness has the tendency to focus on disturbance."[11] Pain, illness, injury, disease, etc. are all significant "disturbances." It is basic human nature to focus on them, talk about them, and worse, incessantly worry about them. It's part of our survival instinct. Problem is, it didn't disconnect when we stopped fleeing *T. rex*.

When dealing with chronic conditions, your mind can get stuck questioning: *How can I prevent another flare-up? How can I avoid pain? If this condition gets worse, what will happen to me? If I have pasta, will my joints swell? If I stay up late, will I be an emotional wreck tomorrow? If I go for a short walk, will it take a week to recover?*

You can't control the way your life works out or what happens to you, your health, or your world, but you're not helpless. In fact, you have a superpower: you can control how you perceive, frame, and react to your reality. Just as your every negative thought takes you further into depression and grief, every positive thought, word, or reaction takes you one step further toward contentment, joy, and well-being. Step by step, you're manifesting your future life for better or worse—and you have the power to choose better!

In nature, the spider uses only materials from within her body to construct her strong, resilient web, which is her world. Like the spider, we too can create a world of powerful medicine using our minds. You don't need a guru or special equipment. You have access to the best possible healer for *you* in the whole wide world: your Inner Healer. S/he's on duty 24/7, free of charge.

With daily discipline, your mind will become your medicine and help heal you.

Shifting to the Thriving Mindset

There are only a few things you really can control:

1) Your thoughts

2) Your words

3) Your emotional reactions

Your thoughts, words, and emotional reactions have power, like magnets. They can be aspirational intentions or curses under your breath. What you think about, talk about, and emote about, you bring about. *Why give more power to negative circumstances? Why not use your circumstances as opportunities to rewire your brain for healing? Why not manifest something positive?*

The good news is, in every moment we can choose our thoughts, words, and reactions. It's as simple as shifting our attention somewhere—anywhere—else (the more positive, the better). It doesn't make the health issue go away, of course. But it will give you relief. So when you catch yourself going on and on in a downward spiral, note it (acknowledge it), and choose something different.

Thoughts, words, and reactions lie behind your actions, which accumulate to create your life and future. By extension, if we can control our unproductive negative thoughts, words, and reactions, we can aim our actions at a more positive, healing future. When we pay attention to our thoughts, words, and reactions, we effectively rewire our brains for maximal healing. That is life-changing.

If we look closer, we see our thoughts become "things"—not necessarily things we can see and feel, but the thoughts, feelings, and even experiences that shape our lives for good or ill. It's the Law of Attraction, known by wise wo/men for centuries. Many have built their lives upon positive visualization, intention setting, vision questing, and so on to attract their desired outcome.

Your attitude becomes your reality and your way of living in this world. *What do you believe? Do you believe you're being pun-*

ished in some way? Or do you believe your health condition may lead you to your life purpose?

When we change our minds, we change our thoughts, words, and reactions to meet what life throws at us—and we change our world. This is called *metanoia*.[12]

Exercise

So, how exactly do you change your mind? We'll do a deeper dive in Chapter 7, "Change Your Mind," but you can begin now with this exercise.

- First, **set your intention** to harness the power of your thoughts, words, and emotional reactions to transform your healing.

- **Become aware of what you're thinking**. A new research study on the human brain suggests the average person typically has more than six thousand thoughts per day.[13] *What are you thinking? Is it positive? Negative?*

- **Release what's wrong**, as it only perpetuates the issue. *What you resist persists*, as they say. The problem you're resisting is actually strengthened by your resistance. What you focus on will be amplified. Negative thoughts are destructive and can send you into a downward spiral of judgment, blame, and disease. Don't give energy to what's wrong in your life. Feel and release any negative or unproductive energy.

- **Amplify the good stuff**. I'm not suggesting you sugarcoat the bad stuff, nor am I advocating fake positivity, but we can't experience the good unless we give it our attention. Focus on what's good, what's working, and what you're able to do. Like a magnet, you'll attract more of it.

- **Shift your perspective** from *disabled* to *able*. From *confinement* to *cocooning*. From *isolation* to *transformation*. It's all in how you reframe it. Someone complains, "One damn thing after another." My outlook is "one adventure after another." Befriend your dragons, don't damn them.

- **Replace "I should" and "I have to" with "I wish to."** It's a subtle shift in energy and intent from being trapped or powerless to being empowered and having agency.

- **Modulate emotional reactions**. Jill Bolte Taylor shares, "When a person has a reaction to something in their environment, there's a 90-second chemical process that happens; any remaining emotional response is just the person choosing to stay in that emotional loop."[14] From a neurological standpoint, beyond that 90 seconds we have a choice about whether we let it go or choose to hold onto it. Choose something positive.

- **Manage expectations**. In other words, don't place unreasonable expectations on yourself given your health condition. This only sets you up for frustration and failure. I don't suggest you give up caring or trying or give up hope. Aim realistically, give it your best, and let go of attachment to a particular (or perfect) outcome.

- **Strive for lightness of being, playfulness of spirit**. If you cultivate this in daily life, then in difficult times, you can find your way back there.

Try this for a few weeks and observe how your health and life change for the better as a result.

This work requires only two disciplines: awareness and tenacity. Speaking from decades of experience, while this is simple, it requires consistent effort. It's so easy for us to obsess about our problems. It takes willpower and intent to focus on positive possibilities. Make it a daily habit with consistent effort. Be tenacious. Stick with it. There's more in chapters to come.

The Prize

Now that you're armed with this powerful tool, *why worry endlessly about how bad things are or how badly you feel?* Open yourself up to the infinite possibilities yet to be discovered in this life of uncertainty.

Whatever life throws at us, we do the best we can. We do not need to struggle to swim upstream against life. Go with the flow. It's about acceptance—surrender—letting go (more on that up ahead). We accept whatever outcome arrives as a stepping-stone to growth. This is immensely healing.

Learn to shift from negative to positive, from suffering to possibility. That's where the fun starts and where you begin creating the health and life of your dreams.

5

WHICH WOLF ARE YOU FEEDING?

The words you speak become the house you live in.

—Hafiz

Native American lore gives us a wonderful story worth gold on the healing journey. Long ago, a Navajo grandfather and his grandson were out walking in the woods. The elder told the boy the story of the two wolves.

"Grandson," he said, "there are two wolves inside of me. One wolf is good, generous, and kind. The other wolf is mean, greedy, and angry. The two wolves within me are always fighting."

The boy listened intently and then asked, "But Grandfather, which one will win?"

The grandfather replied, "The one I feed."

Knowing which wolf you feed with your positive or negative thoughts, words, reactions, and choices can help you reduce your suffering.

In every moment you are faced with any choice, ask yourself, *Is this a positive contribution to my overall healing? to my life purpose?* From television, films, and books to food, drink, and friends, everything you do is a choice—including the choice of whether to be intentional about it or not.

As you go through your day, pay attention: *Which wolf am I feeding with my thoughts?* What you feed it today might not seem to matter, but imagine a daily diet of anger, meanness, and self-loathing. *In a year's time, how does your wolf behave? Is that the wolf you aspire to be? A bitter old wolf?*

It takes courage and strength to face our wolves. But you've got this. Start today: feed your good wolf kindness, compassion, self-love, healthy food, uplifting entertainment. We feed our wolves with our thoughts and also with our spoken words. Complaining about your illness feeds the bad wolf; describing healthy outcomes feeds the good wolf. *Which wolf are you feeding with your words?*

Don't give energy to negative outcomes. You don't need to deny that they may happen or that you're worried, just stop focusing on them. Don't talk excessively about them. Wallowing in self-pity or petulance only gives up precious energy that you could spend on healing thoughts. What does it accomplish anyway? Wallowing only prolongs the misery.

Reframe phrases like "it's always something" and "when it rains, it pours" into "it's always something wonderful" or "when it rains, look for rainbows" (or "when it's dark, look for stars"). This is food for the good wolf. Look through a different lens or from a different perspective to see the good in everything, even when at first it looks like bad, scary stuff.

If you need a cathartic outlet for that bad-wolf food, journal about it. Write it down and let it go. An exercise I find helpful is to gather all my worries, write them on a sheet of paper, and toss them into the fireplace, bury them in the backyard, or fold the paper into a boat and sail it down the stream. Let them go. In this way, we can stop talking about them, which stops feeding the negative energy.

You've got new places to go. Speaking negatively about health issues is an anchor holding you back. It's hard to stop talking about something so serious, so all-consuming. But I did. You can too.

Feeding the good wolf means imagining what you hope to be (healthy!), do, and have. Don't even think about what's hiding in the closet or around that next bend. No matter how bad your diagnosis and prognosis, don't dwell on how bad your future might be.

Live fully in this moment. Is there a bright spot in all the pain, sorrow, grief, loss, and longing? Collect your bright spots and string them together like lights; connect them like dots on a map to a brighter future. One foot in front of the other to a better place.

I'll give you an example of one way I hacked my healing energy. Until August 9, 2017, I counted the days since the disc rupture. I even labeled them on my computer calendar: Day 138. Day 139. Day 140. And so on. August 9, 2017, was Day 244—the day I stopped counting. I wasn't better yet, but I realized that by counting the days since the rupture, I was giving energy to the disability instead of giving energy to healing. I was focusing on the bad wolf.

The same principle goes for answering the question "How are you?" It's often the first question people ask. Seems innocent enough, but it's a potential landmine for healing. The key is not to give your condition any energy by discussing it at length. Focus on perfect health instead.

If you've been feeding the bad wolf all this time, don't beat yourself up. Starting today, lovingly feed your good wolf better thoughts, words, and actions.

To heal takes love, kindness, forgiveness, and peace. Feed your wolf that. Just as the sun emerges from the night and can be counted on every day to make darkness into light, you too will emerge from the darkness of health challenges to a place of light and love.

6

IN THIS MOMENT

*To every thing there is a season,
and a time to every purpose under the heaven . . .
a time to heal.*

—Ecclesiastes 3:1–2, KJV

Everything happens at the right time. If we live our lives by the four seasons, we understand that every season has its purpose—everything happens at the right time. In spring, we're reborn like buds peeking through the snow. In summer, we bloom to full vitality. In autumn, we shed what no longer serves us, like the oak shedding her leaves. In winter, we steel ourselves against the cold, going inward, finding light and warmth, gestating something new that may bud in the spring. So the seasonal cycle goes.

*Only with winter-patience can we bring
the deep-desired, long-awaited spring.*
—Anne Morrow Lindbergh

Life and the healing journey mirror seasonal changes. We can move from thriving and full vitality one day . . . to letting go of what we can no longer do . . . to then marshaling all our resources to get through the dark winter of our soul . . . only to recover and be revitalized like spring.

Remember that you, like the seasons, are in the flow of time. Everything happens in divine timing. Your illness or injury happened at the right time and for a reason in your life's journey and purpose. I know this is tough medicine to take, but if you can stop the cycle of suffering by getting in sync, it's possible to walk over the threshold to thriving.

Here is one of my favorite affirmations (more on affirmations later):

Everything I need comes to me in divine timing.

Healing can mean waiting. It's a test of patience unless we choose to view this holding pattern as we would the waiting for a bud to blossom, carrots to grow in the earth, fruit to ripen to juicy sweetness, a fetus to be born, or sun to rise. We know we cannot rush these things. The caterpillar in the chrysalis only emerges when it's fully ready to be a butterfly. It takes the time that's necessary—not a moment more or less.

Everything happens at the right time, including your healing.

> All shall be well, and all shall be well,
> and all manner of thing shall be well.
> —Lady Julian of Norwich

Uncertainty has enormous, thrilling power. In a moment of uncertainty, anything is possible. What could happen if you were to pivot from seeing your health crisis through a lens of disaster to seeing it as a new season with its own challenges and opportunities? Perhaps this health setback came into your life to open a door to personal and spiritual growth—a door you might not have seen or walked through had you been scurrying around at your normal breakneck pace of life in our hectic, too-fast world. Perhaps your health crisis is the way God, Source, Great Spirit, the Universe, Creator, Goddess, or your Higher Power (whatever you believe) got your attention.

If you can stop struggling and be open—even welcome uncertainty—you can tap into your body's innate healing ability and also find a silver lining to the purpose of your healing journey within your life's journey within your soul's journey.

We know all too well that in one moment something disastrous can happen to our world. Yet at the same time, in one moment, something wonderful can happen! It's a matter of being able to shift your perspective. Instead of thinking with dread, *It's always something*, or *I just can't catch a break*, start saying, *Something wonderful is about to happen*. Then live your life in full expectation that something wonderful *is* about to happen for you. Imagine what that something wonderful looks like and feels like. Visualize it every day.

Before you know it, at the right time, something better comes out of your healing journey. You'll see. You'll cross the threshold from suffering to thriving.

> One day you finally knew what you had to do, and began.
> —Mary Oliver

In This Moment, Everything Is Okay

> The secret of health for both mind and body is not to mourn
> for the past, worry about the future, or anticipate troubles,
> but to live in the present moment wisely and earnestly.
> — Paramhansa Yogananda

Right now are you living in the moment? If you're ruminating about your suffering or making other plans for when you're "all better" or when *this* happens or when *that's* accomplished, then you're not living the beauty of this moment. You're not fully living your life.

If you can fully embody this moment, perhaps you'll find that right now everything is okay. There have been times in my life when I "had it all" but was in a negative spiral. Yet now, medically compromised, I'm more peaceful, positive, and joyful than ever. Why is that? It correlates directly to the inner work I've been doing:

- Recognizing that, in this present moment, everything is okay.

- Intentionally stringing okay moment after okay moment with the belief that, ultimately, it will all be okay.

- Realizing in a bad moment that *this too shall pass*, and I'll get through it. Living in anticipation of bad moments steals today's peace.

- Living in awareness of and gratitude for the beauty and miracle of life surrounding me.

- Observing the quality of my thoughts, actions, and spoken words.

I decided to fully inhabit the present moment and make intentional choices. Now is the perfect time to create a healing atmosphere of "okay" in your life.

When you're injured, disabled, chronically ill, or struggling with mental illness, it's easy to focus on the pain at its worst or anticipate a dreaded medical procedure or catastrophize the worst possible outcome. The human mind excels at this.

It's important to disengage that muscle and ask, *In this moment, how am I really?* If this present moment is not the worst you've ever felt, then you're doing better, right? Let's find a way to live in this present moment. If this is the worst you've ever felt, my heart goes out to you. Know there are better moments ahead.

This practice may feel funny or fake at first, and that's okay. Once during a particularly rough patch when I fell into catastrophizing, my dear friend Carolyn urged me, "Whatever you need to do to trick yourself to be in this moment is what you need to do." She was right. Worrying wasn't helping. I believed in the deeper truth that everything would be okay, so I had to play little mind games with myself to be able to get around the worry to affirm my deeper belief.

Through this process of discernment, I discovered that when I can enter into a moment of stillness, I'm really okay. I'm not wheelchair-bound, for instance, and my pain is manageable. I feel grateful and breathe in relief. I aim to live in this moment without ruminating about painful ones or living in anticipatory fear of suffering. In this moment, I can see light, hopes, dreams. Tomorrow will work itself out. I'll be okay, no matter what unfolds. I trust in that, reminding myself often of the following:

Be here in this moment where everything is okay.
Just for today, live in an expansive space of peace.
Recognize the good, pain-free moments as precious—painful ones as transitory.
Embody the winning attitude that you can overcome your health crisis with grace.

You're going to be okay.
How will you benefit from this mindset shift?

- It will transform your life.
- It will improve your capacity to heal.
- Your outlook on life will be more positive.
- You'll become more intentional about your life and purpose on this earth.
- You'll have more compassion for yourself and others.
- You'll feel good, even when your body doesn't.

- Things that happen in the world, or things people say, won't "hook" you.
- You'll be less likely to spiral downward into despair or tumble down the elevator shaft of depression.[15]
- In other words, you'll find inner peace.

> You never realize how strong you are
> until being strong is the only choice you have.
> —Bob Marley

7
CHANGE YOUR MIND

*Change the way you look at things
and the things you look at will change.*

—Dr. Wayne Dyer

Your health crisis will reveal your mind and true nature. How do you react to bad days? To agonizing pain? To an unpleasant medical procedure or another troubling diagnosis?

Bad moments needn't drown our minds in negativity nor wreck our entire day, month, year, or life. And they won't if we don't allow bad moments to stick to our hearts and minds, taking up residence there. What if you could change your mind about them and find the healing outcome there?

Abracadabra

Our thoughts and words have vibrational energy and power. Remember being a kid and saying the magic incantation "abracadabra"? What have we been talking about except the ways in which we really can use our thoughts and words to change reality? Humans are gifted with the amazing magical ability to control our words and thoughts, and through our intentional selection of them, we can curate our futures.

If you're thinking about negative outcomes 24/7, you're dreaming the wrong dream. You're giving energy to the negative outcome. Once you shift your thoughts and intentions to the positive, imagine your dream clearly, and feel the outcome, you're on your way to dreaming a new world for yourself.

Over the past couple of decades, I've put this principle into daily practice—it has changed my life. But never has the power of thoughts and words been more transformational than through the difficult years of incapacitation. Given how utterly miserable and limiting my condition was year after year, I should have been depressed. Yet this has been one of the most joyful, creatively fertile, highly productive, contented times of my life!

What's the secret? We can train our brains to see the positive by reframing. Just as you create any good habit or skill, reframing takes practice.

Reframing

On a bad day, I work hard to accept that a bad moment just happened and banish any negative thoughts that hang around. I don't let the bad stuff take up residence in my heart by ruminating on it.

Then I look on the bright side. Yes, even if you're completely bedridden as I was, there can be a bright side. We can talk about how unfair it is or we can find a positive outcome or new opportunity presented by the setback. We can reframe it.

My internal dialogue might go something like this:

- **Bad day or unpleasant medical procedure**—*This too shall pass. Tomorrow will be better. I'm grateful to be alive another day.* Then I really inhabit that feeling, visualizing all the wonderful things for which I'm grateful. I focus on feeling a sense of accomplishment about how far I've come, and I celebrate the little victories. *Breathe deep. It's over now. Hit the reset button. Let go of the fear and anxiety. I'll feel better tomorrow. I'm grateful to live in an age of medical miracles!* I'm hopeful about tomorrow.

- **Setback**—Instead of, *Oh, damn you, knee!* (when the meniscus tears) I say, *Thank you, my beautiful body, for getting me so well along my life's journey—I love you and will take care of us.* It's disempowerment vs. empowerment.

My barn having burned down, I can now see the moon.
—Mizuta Masahide

Change Your Habits of Mind

Choosing our thoughts and words with care enables us to change our habitual mind, that is, the human mind's habit of catastrophizing, worrying, and otherwise running amok, speeding down the slippery slope of spiraling negative thoughts.

There's a funny thing about thoughts of fear and painful experiences: they get stuck in a loop. That's what we do, quite unconsciously, with our painful feelings, paralyzing fears, and hurtful thoughts. We hold onto them deep inside where they constrict our hearts and emotions. They take up precious space where we could grow beautiful creations.

You can disrupt this by being intentional: *What am I attracting? Is it positive or negative?*

The mind doesn't need to be a runaway train or a loop of angst. It can be taught to focus on transforming negative challenges into positive opportunities. It is possible to simply observe the thoughts, fears, and feelings, and let them sail past without attaching to your heart.

Here it is in the simplest terms:

- Shine the spotlight of awareness on the positive change you're seeking.

- Hit the reset button immediately upon recognizing a negative thought.
- Replace the negative with your dream of a better outcome.

Let's take a deeper dive into how we change our minds. With daily concerted effort, this five-step formula will yield transformational results. It's time-tested through the centuries.

STEP ONE: CULTIVATE AWARENESS

The deep silence of the void is where the magic happens. A quiet, aware mind is a blank canvas waiting for you to create upon it.

Be mindful of negative thoughts. They steal your peace. Weed out those negative thoughts before they put down deep roots and strangle the blossoms of more positive thoughts.

> Happiness is a butterfly, which, when pursued, is always just beyond your grasp, but which, if you will sit down quietly, may come and alight on you.
> —Author Unknown

Vigilantly observe your thoughts throughout the day. Pay attention to your monkey mind, the endless stream of chatter in your brain. Through meditation, intentional thought, breathwork, and such, we can observe our mind and in so doing cultivate a new habit.

Michael Singer explains how meditation helps us turn back toward the outer world: "As you pull back into the consciousness, the world ceases to be a problem. It's just something you're watching."[16] In other words, your health challenges cease to be *problems*, per se, and become things to which you've assigned the label *problem*. Just observe them.

Step Two: Forgive and Let Go

When negative thoughts linger, visualize them as water and watch them flow away. You cannot grasp water—it flows. Turn your negative thoughts into water, forgive them, let them wash away, and let them go.

For example, I used this technique to dispel recurring anger at the people who were irresponsible with my health: the personal trainer who was well aware of my back issue yet insisted I do contraindicated twisty exercises with weights (it led to the first disc rupture), the physical therapist who applied unnecessary pressure to my spine during a stretch (a second rupture), the chiropractor who did a hard adjustment despite my request not to (thus the most severe rupture).

I worked on forgiving them as I visualized them drifting away from me on a boat down the river. It cleared space in my mind that made room for visualizing healing.

Step Three: Shift Focus and Reframe

Once we observe the problems our mind has identified, we can reframe them from *problems* to *opportunities*. My health *problem* has offered me myriad *opportunities* for fulfillment and happiness. Now I focus on that.

Remember, in every moment, we have a choice. For instance, changing your mind requires choosing your focus. You can choose to admire glorious blooms or be consumed by cursing the weeds.

Also intentionally focus your actions: *What are you subscribing to that's negative? News, social media, negative or toxic people?* Try to minimize those. I curate my world in a very intentional way. No gratuitously violent entertainment; I prefer uplifting, humorous entertainment because it helps me heal. I love to listen to inspiring stories of those who overcame obstacles. They cultivate hope.

Intentionally let go of negative thoughts/actions and choose positive ones. Plant them like seeds. Water them daily. Tend to them like a garden—be laser-focused on cultivating the healing ones.

I practice this awareness while meditating and throughout the day: in the shower, in conversations with others, cooking dinner, etc. Ever-present awareness of mind means being ever vigilant. Every day. Every moment. Try to hold that focus out there in the world—at work, at the store, with friends and family. Watch your world and your health transform.

Step Four: Take Aim

For centuries, wise ones have said "Thoughts become things." If you focus on how small and debilitating your life has become, that will be your lived experience. Like a magnet, you'll attract more of that into your life. Yet the opposite is also true: when you focus on the good—the opportunity or blessing in your circumstance—you'll attract more positive experiences.

It's like driving a car, aiming an arrow, or playing any sport. Where we focus is the direction we go. Be an arrow—your thoughts, words, and actions are your powerful bow. Take aim at peace, happiness, and the future you wish to create. Let your thoughts, words, and actions propel you there. Our minds are hardwired to look at the negative. What's called our "reptilian mind" will scout for dangers even if most of the worst dangers aren't our realities anymore, and respond with *fight-flight-freeze* as survival mechanisms.

Don't unintentionally aim at the place you don't wish to go by continuing to think, worry, or talk about what's wrong in your life. Aim for the good stuff.

Your thoughts—good or bad—are seeds of intention. They need the water and sunshine of positivity to blossom and thrive. Be careful of planting seeds of doubt, fear, negative outcomes, etc. or your garden will flourish with invasive weeds. Don't deny the negative like an ostrich with your head in the sand. Survey the whole landscape and scan everything, good and bad, but don't dwell on the negative or let it hook you into going down the rabbit hole, or worse, falling down the elevator shaft into the abyss.

There's magic in setting an intention. It begins moving your energy in the direction of your dreams. It couldn't be simpler:

- Take a few deep breaths.
- Quiet your mind.
- Tune into your awareness (body and mind).
- Visualize what you wish to manifest, crystal clear, and state your intention.
- Feel it deeply. How will you feel when it manifests? Embody that feeling.
- Be ready to receive it.
- *Believe* it is on the way, and feel deep gratitude, for it is.

It's super important to believe with all your heart that your dream is coming true. This is why a placebo works—people who take it believe it will cure them. When we fully believe what we manifest will come to fruition, it will. *What do you believe?*

STEP FIVE: THE CHANGED LIFE

With practice your new mind will habitually observe your thoughts, allowing the good ones to take hold and releasing negative ones. It took me years to learn this, but today, it's my practice. All the work to cultivate this intentional state of mind has been transformational. The precious result is living in a perpetual state of peace, contentment, happiness, gratitude, and openness. In this state, no matter what other people say or think of you, no matter what is going on in the world or your own life, you'll have an unshakable sense of being grounded.

But I don't want to make it sound like all that work was one long struggle *in addition* to my physical pain. Rather, I've found the process itself profoundly euphoric. Like everything, results are incremental. It's like learning to dance, painting your house, or planting a garden. Start with baby steps. Once you've experienced it, you won't want to go back to being a slave to your monkey mind, the runaway thoughts chattering in your head.

Now I won't let anything jeopardize this state. It's worth every minute of weeding out the unproductive thoughts and remaining ever vigilant to maintain this optimal consciousness.

When you heal yourself, you heal the world. Start with your own mind.

> Where we put our awareness, and for
> how long, maps our destiny.
> —Dr. Joe Dispenza

Choose Joy

> Everything can be taken from a man but one thing: the last of the human freedoms—to choose one's attitude in any given set of circumstances, to choose one's own way.
> —Viktor Frankl

The above quotation inspires me. If Frankl could choose to be positive while surviving the Holocaust's inhumanity, then I too can choose my attitude, no matter how terrible my circumstances.

We always have a choice. Certainly, we can choose to wallow in a loop of suffering, or we can choose a different path. The hard truth is you might be ill, injured, pain-ridden, or in the hospital or hospice for your remaining days.

So why not decide—right now—to choose joy for the rest of your days no matter what happens in the world or your personal life, whether your health gets better or worse?

Focus on what brings you joy. You've heard "happiness is an inside job." We must choose in every moment to find some sense of happiness that bubbles up from within. We won't find it externally.

Anger and happiness cannot coexist. Neither can bitterness and contentment or misery and peace.

Heaven or hell here on earth—it's your choice. It is hugely empowering to realize that, in every moment, the choice is yours. Choose something and make it good. In every moment, choose to find the most joyful way through this healing journey. By building moments of joy, we build a lifetime of joy regardless of health crises.

Commit to unconditional joy, no matter what happens. Let go of expectations and parameters. Choosing joy rewires our brains with their sparkling neuroplasticity (something I encourage you to learn more about).

Joy never leaves us. It may get overshadowed by fear, stress, and busyness, or we feel as though it has taken flight, abandoning us forever. But you can always call it back again.

> There is no value in life except what you choose to place upon it, and no happiness in any place except what you bring to it yourself.
> —Lin Yutang

PART 3

Preparing Your Mind and Spirit

> When we no longer know what to do
> we have come to our real work and . . .
> when we no longer know which way to go,
> we have begun our real journey.
>
> —Wendell Berry

8
THERE WILL BE TEARS

> Where there is sorrow there is holy ground.
>
> —Oscar Wilde

When you're sick or injured, loss can hit you like a ton of bricks.

When my disc ruptured so disastrously, I lost my health, my work, my mobility. I lost my ability to go out and socialize. I lost a couple of friendships. I lost my dreams. My studio—my happy place in which I wrote poetry, created art, and rehearsed music—was abandoned for five years and looks like an archeological dig, dust covering now-distant memories.

Severe disease/injury can be like a death: we grieve the "me" we used to be. We experience all the stages of grief. When we lose a loved one, it leaves a hole in our heart, a deep, aching, disorienting loss. Loss resulting from a health crisis is a lot like that. We lose so many things we enjoy and that are good for us, and the resulting grief can be deeply painful.

For a time, grieving the life, mobility, and freedom I'd lost and the future "me" I'd planned to be was devastating. I wondered, *Will this grief ever end?* Grief has layers like an onion; when you think you're done, there's another layer. The grief may always be with you, but it's essential to walk the road of grief for as long as it takes to heal.

The people in your life understand you will grieve, but they may expect your grief to last only a month or a year. Don't worry about them. Grief takes as long as it needs to. What it boils down to is the more deeply we love—a hobby, athletic ability, or health—and the more passionately we live, the more devastating the loss and the longer the grieving process.

Loss can be a long leg of your journey; it's okay to plumb the depths of it. I remember fondly when I used to be able to dance with abandon, swim, walk after work along a forest path, and jump in my car with my camera for an adventure. I remember when I was able to play flute and perform on weekends, paint at my easel, travel abroad, and throw dinner parties. I still grieve these losses. But at the same time, I'm grounded deeply in acceptance that those days are gone, and I hold hope that new terrain to explore is on the horizon.

Illness teaches us that loss of one sort can be a gain of another kind if viewed through the proper lens of acceptance. It's about looking for the silver lining and being transformed in the process. Even in great loss, it's possible to find beauty and joy.

We don't arrive at this space of acceptance overnight. We must face our loss, fully embody it, and honor it. "The way in is the way out" is the pithy version of this, and it's particularly true here.

Healing from Loss

To heal from loss, we cannot turn away from, numb, or bury it. Facing loss can be a springboard for growth. This transformation following a traumatic event is called post-traumatic growth.

Elizabeth Kübler-Ross described the five stages of grief: denial, anger, bargaining, depression, and acceptance.[17] If you're facing a major health crisis, terminal or not, you'll likely experience these stages. They can be transformational in a positive way. You can't spell *blossom* without *loss*. How fitting, because when we allow ourselves to work through the grief of our loss we can truly blossom. Many people, myself included, are transformed by loss and go on to blossom and build fulfilling lives.

Writing about organizations that grew exponentially, Salim Ismail reports, "Google recently demonstrated that its best employees were not Ivy League students, but rather young people who had experienced a big loss in their lives and had been able to transform that experience into growth. According to Google, deep personal loss has resulted in employees who are more humble and open to listening and learning."[18]

Think about that. Even in a business context, a loss can be turned into professional growth.

When everything is taken away, the light shines through and illuminates a new way. Loss re-routes your life journey and propels your growth. So take the time you need to grieve this unexpected, unwanted transition you've found yourself in, but don't be defined by it. Ask yourself these questions:

- What might be the silver lining, the light shining through the darkness?
- What new road do I see?
- What new adventure might I incubate?

No matter how dark things seem today, you'll find a way through to a new way of being. If a new path is not immediately visible (it rarely is, early on), keep looking. Take time to contemplate these questions and answers will reveal themselves. At some point, you'll be able to decide what comes next and step into your destiny with bravery and hope.

When I posed those questions to myself, I found the silver lining: opportunities to explore new interests and write more. The new road before me, shining brightly, is this book you're reading— the contemplations and wisdom I've incubated through this decades-long healing journey. The suffering

I endured hasn't been for naught. It's hugely rewarding for me to be of service in this way.

Anticipatory Grief

In addition to grieving losses, we humans tend to grieve our anticipated futures. Grief experts call this *anticipatory grief*, that is, the grief we feel in anticipation of some suffering or loss we foresee. We felt this anticipatory grief in spring 2020 when the pandemic ravaged our communities and we went into lockdown.[19] We all had this sense that things were going to get worse; we were losing something by staying home, and we were going to lose even more.

Anticipatory grief has been a challenge for me regarding my physical health. My spine is progressively deteriorating and has been for decades. I can't help but think ahead to my future, and so I've learned firsthand the surest road to misery is catastrophizing about what my mobility might be ten years hence.

The surest path to peace, however, is to be in the present moment, grateful for good health today. The Toolkit will help you with this. I practice daily to thwart anticipatory grief before it takes root.

No conversation about loss is complete without mentioning the ultimate loss: death. If you or a loved one are near death, the skills I share here can certainly help, but I encourage you to explore the many resources specifically designed to help make walking this part of the path more conscious, comfortable, and peace-filled.[20]

> Cry. Forgive. Learn. Move on.
> Let your tears water the seeds of your future happiness.
> —Steve Maraboli

No Shame in Tears

On the healing journey, there will be tears—when you're given the scary diagnosis, in pain, overwhelmed, fearing uncertainty, or mourning the loss of your "old life" and dreams of what you might have become.

There's no shame in tears. It's more than okay to cry—tears can be good medicine. Tears open the door to calm and help us facilitate acceptance of our circumstances. Scientific studies demonstrate that tears can release pain, stress, overwhelm, anxiety, and hurt.

We must protect our physical body by processing emotions and filtering our mental ramblings. So if you need to cry, here's your permission slip. Don't let emotions fester, stagnate, and become baggage. Feel them fully, then let the emotions pass through you—like air through a screen—without getting stuck and harming your health.

It's liberating. Easier said than done, of course, but it only requires a mindset shift and determination.

If you're struggling with overwhelming grief, remember it's not a sign of weakness to seek the help of a mental health professional.

> The most beautiful people we have known are those who have known defeat, known suffering, known struggle, known loss, and have found their way out of the depths.
> —Elizabeth Kübler-Ross

9

A STAMPEDE OF HORSES: PAIN

> The easy days ahead of you will be easy. It is the hard days—the times that challenge you to your very core—that will determine who you are. You will be defined not just by what you achieve, but by how you survive.
>
> —Sheryl Sandberg

If you're in relentless pain, know you're not alone. According to the CDC, "In 2019, 20.4% of [US] adults [50 million] had chronic pain and 7.4% of adults had chronic pain that frequently limited life or work activities (referred to as high impact chronic pain) in the past 3 months."[21] That's one in five Americans having chronic pain. That means there's a strong chance someone you know lives with chronic pain, whether they've shared that with you or not.

But we're not good, as a society, at talking about chronic pain. This book is my contribution toward changing that.

Understanding Pain

Pain is an alarm—your body's signal to your brain warning you something is wrong. There are two types of pain: acute and chronic. Acute pain is "of sudden onset and is usually the result of a clearly defined cause such as an injury. Acute pain resolves with the healing of its underlying cause." By contrast, chronic pain "persists for weeks or months and is usually associated with an underlying condition, such as arthritis."[22] Some kinds of chronic pain can be resolved while others must be managed.

Severe pain can be urgent, demanding, and at times, all-consuming—beyond your threshold and completely debilitating. Pain does all of the following:

- affects ability to work, concentrate, walk, exercise, and socialize
- limits ability to perform everyday tasks like dressing, bathing, cooking, cleaning
- interferes with relationships, causing social isolation that can lead to depression and serious health conditions[23]
- causes sleep deprivation
- triggers irritability and overwhelm
- undermines our ability to enjoy life
- causes premature aging

In other words, pain can be life-altering.

Pain Changes Our Demeanor

My chronic pain never lets up. Even with meds, I'm never not in pain. It's inescapable. Since chronic pain entered my life decades ago, I've felt like two different people. On the one hand, there's who I think of as the "regular" me—the active, hopeful person who I've been seeing less of as years go by. When my pain is controlled, I can inhabit this self enough to focus on my hopes and dreams.

The "other" me is wracked with pain—broken, tearful, writhing, hyperventilating, agitated, unable to do the most basic tasks (stand, sit, walk, sleep). The pain is either peripheral nerve pain, back pain, and/or sciatica. I have pain even on a good day, and I slowly deteriorate as the day progresses and pain dials up higher. I constantly juggle my day to accommodate my pain level with bed rest. When pain is severe, this suffering me crowds out any thoughts of "regular" me.

Sometimes pain can be so severe we're entirely incapable of doing anything but breathe, and even this can be unbearable. Pain is like a stampede of runaway horses. We need to rein it in or else we lose control and it overruns us.

It can be a vicious cycle: wake up in pain > get to work > experience stress > accelerating pain > more stress > more and more pain > fear > anxiety > painsomnia > repeat. Sound familiar?

This cycle affects social life. Because our energy and pain ebb and flow from day to day, hour to hour, and cannot be predicted, we lose the ability to make firm commitments. If we do make plans, we end up breaking them or rescheduling again and again. Even with the best intentions, we become an unreliable friend and, over time, find ourselves increasingly isolated.

Years ago, in a long pain cycle that included severe cyclical Raynaud's peripheral nerve pain on top of chronic, severe spinal pain, I considered ending it all. Nerve pain in my feet and hands eclipsed the debilitating back pain, unimaginable as that was. I knew they were both progressively worsening conditions. I was in a state of despair. I wasn't hopeless because I was immobile, disabled, and living my life from bed. I was hopeless because of the relentless, off-the-charts pain.

But then I saw the daffodils peeking their heads above the snow, a reminder of spring and better times ahead. I held onto hope, recognizing that at some point the pain would be in the rearview mirror. *This too shall pass.*

Perhaps you can relate to this. I needed the pain to stop. Knowing I had suicide as an option actually provided some relief, assuring me I had some last measure of control. For me, having seen the endless suffering of those who've lost a loved one to suicide, I couldn't go through with it. But that doesn't mean the thought doesn't cross my mind.

This is a good place to say that if you feel suicide is becoming more than just a fantasy of escape, please get help immediately.

Right now, it's difficult for me to imagine a life without pain, but I know I must never lose hope. Choosing to live, I accept pain as part of life. Thankfully, human brains are hardwired to forget past pain (like childbirth). What's more, our pain threshold (measured on a subjective scale of zero to ten) shifts as we experience pain levels that break our previous records. What would have sent me racing to the emergency room decades ago is now my "normal." You can live a full, joyful life despite pain.

How to Cope with Pain

For many of us, managing pain is a full-time job. Much energy goes toward keeping pain below our threshold, the point beyond which we can no longer endure and push through it. You can survive that unbearable monster pain with grace and find contentment on the other side.

We can try to deal with pain in four ways:

- ignore it
- distract ourselves from it
- make adaptations to our lives
- explore it and learn something from it

Sometimes, if it's mild, pain can be ignored. However, if it's severe and chronic, that's impossible. Distraction—in the form of work, TV/movies, music, games, sex, etc.—isn't effective either.

To minimize pain and prevent flare-ups, we can make adaptations to our daily lives. Adaptations, a.k.a. work-arounds, are as unlimited as your imagination. It's important to find adaptations that help you minimize your pain so you can thrive.

Severe pain can be so loud and prolonged we cannot hear our body's wisdom. It helps to turn toward our pain and sit with it. Explore it. Learn what it's telling us. We can benefit from our bodies' wisdom.

Over the years, I've found a number of pain tools. Let's begin with traditional pain management.

First Things First
The science around pain is evolving quickly. Be sure to speak with your doctor.

- **Consider Over-The-Counter (OTC) Products**

    The anti-inflammatory Voltaren gel is now nonprescription. I've used it with excellent results for knee pain and joint pain in my hands. Magnesium spray or cream is soothing for soft tissue issues such as torn muscles and tendons, as are Epsom salts baths (it's the magnesium content). OTC lidocaine and thermal patches may help. Arnica is good for bumps and bruises. Consider trying CBD balms as well. Capsaicin and essential oils might be appropriate for some issues. Ask your pharmacist what's right for you.

- **Medications**

    When pain is beyond your threshold, consult your doctor for advice on anti-inflammatory meds, pain blockers, muscle relaxers, cortisone or hyaluronic gel injections (viscosupplements), pain meds, etc. My pain management cocktail consists of Voltaren (anti-inflammatory), amitriptyline (early generation depression med that blocks pain signal to brain), pregabalin (nerve pain blocker), steroids when needed, and pain medication for breakthrough pain.

- **Act Fast**

    Doctors will tell you to jump on pain relief quickly, before it gets out of control. I'd add, hit it with everything you can: heat and/or ice, breathwork, massage, or whatever is relevant to your condition (see below).

Other Techniques
When traditional interventions aren't enough—or if you seek to avoid/minimize prescription meds—the techniques below might help take the edge off your pain so you can hear your inner wisdom, the embodied intelligence of your body, and tune in to what your body needs at this moment. (There's more in Part 6.) Like most things in life, real results come with steady practice. If these resonate with you, consider making them a habit.

- **Breathing**

    When pain is severe, muscles tighten and breathing becomes clenched and shallow. As a result, injured/diseased parts don't receive enough oxygen. Tension makes pain worse. Research demonstrates that pain can diminish with deep, healing breaths. Conscious, full breathing can slow the mind and calm us when panicked by our pain level. It alleviates muscle tightness, which may help dial pain down a notch. Breathing brings blood flow to the painful area, which is vital to healing.

- **Body Scan for Deep Relaxation and Relief**

    Chapter 36, "The Guided Journey," has more details on this technique. During the body scan exercise, imagine breathing directly into the painful area (e.g., hip). Visualize your breath entering that specific area and oxygenating all the cells there. Invite the pain to leave as it no longer serves you. For some types of pain, this is effective. Others not so much. Give it a try.

- **Athletic Listening**

  Listen deeply and give your full attention to your inner wisdom (a.k.a. intuition, gut instinct). What language is your body "speaking" pain? (Or is it tension, fatigue, fear, anxiety, nausea, headaches?) What is the pain trying to tell you (*don't do this movement or activity, or do more of that: rest, relax, unplug, massage*, etc.)? Where is your threshold? Is it ten minutes of walking? Five minutes of standing? An hour of sitting in a chair? If your injury/condition gets worse with activity, your body is warning you. Pay attention to that. Keep a journal to help track what makes your pain better/worse.

- **Adaptation**

  Once you know your threshold, honor it by taking action, doing more/less of whatever works for you. Then ponder this: *For optimal health, is there a better way of doing things?* Figure out work-arounds. Purchase adaptive items to help. You'll discover everything from devices to help you put on socks to braces for most body parts, special support pillows, bolsters, etc.

  (For spinal conditions, I've found these items invaluable in reducing discomfort and enabling me to have a somewhat more normal life: cutout seat cushions, lumbar back support, a Lunix LX5 four-piece orthopedic bed wedge memory foam pillow set, ergonomically adaptive computer desk, voice assistance devices, massagers, braces for wrist, back, knee)

  Adaptations help you move things off the list of activities you cannot do and onto the list of things you can still do if you apply a little creativity. After considerable searching, I even found a flute support stand to balance the end of my flute without torqueing my spine. I cannot hold a flute otherwise. With it, I can play for ten minutes, which is better than nothing. I've structured my life around adaptations, which have given me part of my life back. Never give up on finding adaptations. Leave no stone unturned in your search for relief.

- **Gentle Movement and Heat**

  For some health issues, movement is a benefit, while for others, it can be damaging. Listen to your body (and your medical team!) on this one. Consider gentle movement: yoga/chair yoga, massage, myofascial release, acupuncture/acupressure/trigger points, and stretching. Unlike stretching before going for a run, gentle stretching can be quite helpful for dialing down pain from sciatica, for example.[24] Heat expands blood vessels, thereby invigorating the painful area(s) with oxygen essential for easing traumatized muscles and vital for healing in general.

- **Limit Movement**

  If your condition is worsened by motion, speak to your doctor or physical therapist about whether intentional immobilization will help avoid escalating pain and further damage. As difficult as it is, I've structured my entire life around limiting activity to what I can do from bed in order to manage extreme pain. This is what I call living below your pain threshold. If we overdo it, we'll most surely pay for it with increased pain and longer recovery time.

- **Reduce Inflammation**

  Inflammation is often the root source of pain and can be like a runaway train unless we actively tackle it.

Research demonstrates that instead of, or in addition to, anti-inflammatory meds, numerous effective avenues are possible. If appropriate for your condition, ice the inflamed area. Take a warm Epsom salts bath (high in magnesium) to ease muscle/joint pain (add organic essential oils of blue tansy, lavender, eucalyptus, chamomile, rosemary, or yarrow for further benefit).

Remove inflammatory foods from your diet: sugar, wheat/gluten, nightshades, lectins, dairy, and acidic foods and drinks (such as coffee, soft drinks, alcohol, processed foods, etc., are linked to numerous health problems and cause inflammation). When your body becomes less inflamed, pain lessens, and healing can begin. (See Chapter 16: "Super Sleuthy You.") After beginning an anti-inflammatory diet a couple of decades ago, my asthma has all but disappeared and my arthritis pain evaporated.

- **Reduce Nerve Pain**

One of the worst pains to endure, nerve pain can feel like a thousand burning hot needles piercing your skin. Pregabalin works for me. However, I've found organic essential oils (such as Frankincense & Myrrh Neuropathy Oil), applied topically, can reduce pain a notch. While plant-based essential oils might sound a bit "out there" to you, their healing benefits have been touted for centuries. Today they are a billion-dollar industry and confirmed by scientific research.

The best medicine, of course, is to avoid flare-ups in the first place. Know your triggers. For example, when my work stress is high, the nerve pain flares to unbearable levels. If I consciously reduce my stress, I can minimize flare-ups. You'll find stress reduction techniques in Part 6.

- **Natural Supplements for Pain Relief and Relaxation**

  With spinal/joint issues, I've found my daily multi-collagen complex to be amazing. For five years it has helped to slow the progression of degenerative skeletal/joint conditions and nourishes my body with what it requires to remain strong and healthy. Magnesium, turmeric (2,000 mg), and white willow are three of my go-to supplements for pain. I use arnica for bruises, pain, and soreness of traumatized muscles (e.g., contusion, elongation, strain). Valerian root, ashwagandha, *Rhodiola rosea*, 5-HTP, mucuna, skullcap, and vervain help with overall relaxation and stress relief. The products Inflavonoid Intensive Care and Kaprex help fight inflammation, often the root cause of pain, as mentioned above. Ask your doctor about these as well as CBD oil and medical marijuana.

- **Painsomnia Solutions**

  When we're ill, our bodies require more sleep. Cutting our sleep hours short and powering through tasks when our bodies need rest only prolongs healing time. I devoted Chapter 18, "Bears Do It, Bees Do It," to this important topic. In addition to previously mentioned sleep hygiene and relaxation protocols, DreamWell (melatonin and GABA) and amitriptyline (an early generation depression med with sedative side effects) have enabled me to sleep most of the night. Without these, I slept in twenty-minute jags because of pain disruption. Ask your doctor.

- **Acceptance, Affirmations, Visualization, and Meditation**

  When pain is horrific, you've tried everything, and there's nothing more you can do, then acceptance of your circumstances is better than tormenting yourself with negative thoughts and emotions. I find repeating an acceptance manta ("I am in pain now, and it will pass. It always does.") helps take away my anticipatory fear as I'm bracing for the worst. I remind myself I always come back from this horribly painful place. I *will* feel better. *This too shall pass.* Explore Emotional Freedom Technique (EFT) Tapping, a combination of tapping on certain meridians of the body and stating an affirmation that many people report being helpful in rewiring their neurology. A friend holds a lapis lazuli crystal for pain relief. Experiment.

Without these practices, I'd be in significantly worse pain. Do they relieve all my pain? No. Do they take it down a notch? Yes, definitely. These protocols have enabled me to survive long years of unbearable pain and even the worst moments when pain medications weren't available.

You might experience more pain than I do. If so, I hope you find some relief here. Give it a try. Be sure to stick with it for a while.

Another key factor is a positive attitude. I say more about this in other chapters. Fortunately, I've had the personality and life experiences that allow me to maintain a positive attitude most of the time. I believe wholeheartedly I'll eventually heal, and this helps me make positive self-care choices.

Don't give up hope. We must believe our health condition(s) will get better and our pain will lessen. This belief gets us through the worst days. Those of us who can do this have an easier time of it.

As you make changes in order to manage your pain, you may find some of your adaptations inconvenience others in your life. Be prepared for pushback and stand strong for your own self-care. It's okay to tell others you're in pain and need to do x, y, or z. Do what you need to do to take care of yourself.

The ultimate lesson is (and this applies to all illnesses and injuries) to listen to your body. Listen to the pain. The more aware you become, the more you'll learn from your body. Trust yourself.

THE MIND–BODY CONNECTION

We often think—and some books and medical professionals actually say—that our bodies are betraying us. That's not the case. Our bodies are trying to get our attention. It took me a while to realize my ailing body is not my enemy. It's more like a vulnerable child who needs care, balance, and love.

Let's dive deeper into the notion of exploring pain as a coping mechanism. I know, this sounds scary. Pain is a scary, intense place. We try to avoid it all our lives. However, when we explore the scary places, the body reveals its instruction manual. It's where we find the wisdom to cope and not just survive but thrive.

Much has been written about the mind–body connection, brain therapy, unified whole-brain function, etc. Learn more about them. I'll highlight a couple of approaches.

Jon Kabat-Zinn[25] offers a method of turning toward the pain and getting to know it by asking the following questions:

- What is it telling me?
- How does it change as I observe it?
- What makes it less bad? Worse?

I've found this to be valuable in reducing the fear and dread of pain. Kabat-Zinn also suggests a brilliant method of focusing on the parts of your body that aren't experiencing pain.[26] This is the only form of "distraction" I've found helpful.

No discussion of pain is complete without mentioning that physical and psychological pain go hand in hand. Emotional pain and trauma—experiencing death, divorce, child abuse, sexual abuse, domestic violence, addiction, poverty, community violence—can leave an imprint not only on our minds and emotions but also on our bodies.

In other words, our emotional lives are tied to physical expression. Research by Dr. Gabor Maté shows the correlation between emotions and trauma and the stress-disease connection, or psychoimmunology—the science of interactions between the mind and body.[27] When we suppress anger and other emotions, we suppress our immune system, which may increase the onset of autoimmune and other diseases.

The dissonance between the life you want and the life you have, if left to fester, can create dis-ease. Merle Shain tells us "despair is anger with no place to go, pain that has gone inside and dug in deep, and because the body and the mind are not two separate things but only one, the mind's pain usually shows up somewhere else, so the search for self is a search for health."[28]

>Feelings are signposts.
>—Llyn Roberts

Recognize, feel, and honor your emotions. Process them. Look at them with curiosity: *What are you trying to teach me? What do I need to learn?*

Most importantly, don't allow anger and other emotions to put down roots. Feel sad. Face grief. Address anger. But don't wallow in them.

Know that you have legitimate needs:

- to feel and process your emotions fully
- to live your authentic life
- to say *no* to what isn't authentic or is a compulsive reaction to help others while ignoring your own health needs—or taking rigid responsibility for duty over and above taking care of yourself

What area(s) of your life are you *not* saying no to, to the detriment of your health?

You also need a place to talk about your feelings. Some individuals bottle up, suppress, or deny their true emotions. Science continues to demonstrate that if we suppress emotions, denying our feelings, they can lead to mental and physical "dis-ease" and chronic illness.

If this describes you, consider it a red flag. Take time to connect with and express your feelings (responsibly, of course):

- reach out to your network of friends to speak your needs, share, or ask for help

- express your feelings by journaling

- create art, write a poem, explore movement/dancing, sing, paint, draw, beat a drum

- change your mind by shifting your perspective, possibly from the victim mentality (*something is being done to me*) to empowerment (*I'm being given an opportunity to learn and grow and harvest pearls of wisdom*)

- explore talk therapy with a professional therapist or art therapist

> Let me not beg for the stilling of my pain
> but for the heart to conquer it.
> —Rabindranath Tagore

10

SURVIVING ISOLATION: HOUSEBOUND SHUT-IN TO LIT-UP HOMEBODY

> Isolation is a way to know ourselves.
>
> —Franz Kafka

Okay, so you're homebound and hibernating, and it feels super nourishing . . . until it doesn't. At some point, most of us begin to get cabin fever after prolonged isolation. When there's no end in sight, we become impatient and restless. *Now what?*

Isolation can magnify a hair-trigger tension between feeling safe versus feeling trapped, comfortable versus claustrophobic, and alone versus lonely. It can be challenging to learn to dance with it, but it is possible.

Reframing Isolation

If we begin to look through a different lens, our health crises can provide us with opportunities to explore the riches of solitude that an otherwise active, healthy period of our lives might not permit. As Fenton Johnson tells us, the difficult path can sometimes be the most rewarding, with the grandest vistas and sweetest thrills.[29]

If you're housebound, ask, *How can I reframe this period and channel it into something positive?* Consider some opportunities:

- **A Time of Study**—Would you like to learn something new? A language? A skill? A course of study? A mindfulness practice?

- **A Time of Creativity**—Ask any musician, writer, artist, dancer, or actor and they'll share how alone time is vital to creativity. While artistic pursuits come to mind, you can use your creativity to plan menus for beautiful meals or crafty projects like knitting, jewelry-making, and woodworking.

- **A Time of Dreaming, Planning, or Seed Planting**—You could plan a home improvement project, new business, or garden.

- **A Time of Reading**—It's a great time to explore your favorite authors, art or travel books, the classics, personal development, etc. Ditto for catching up on films.

What new or buried interests are seeking your attention? Follow the meandering thread of your instincts and you'll find deep fulfillment there.

Happy Homebody

I was convalescing in isolation for four years, and just as I was physically able to get out more, *wham*, here comes COVID-19. When pandemic lockdowns occurred, I had an advantage over many people because I already had well-established coping mechanisms for going from housebound shut-in to lit-up homebody.

We'll look at these coping mechanisms under three headings:

- Make your surroundings a healing sanctuary, a place of refuge.
- Create a shrine to healing.
- Create rituals to shift energy, focus your mind, and add meaning, peace, and heightened awareness to your days.

Little tweaks to your environment can propel your capacity to heal, even if you're not shut-in or bedridden. Furthermore, you'll heal better if you feel loved—and self-love made visible through your surroundings and everyday rituals. Create an abundance of love that reflects back on your strength and wellness. The following ideas will get you started.

> We have to love ourselves into the Being we want to become . . . that's what makes us heal and grow.
> —Eileen McKusick

Fashion a Serene Healing Sanctuary, a Place of Refuge

When my disc ruptured, leaving me bedridden 24/7, I urgently needed to mentally escape the pain and complete debilitation. I often did so by recalling happy travels. One day I was reminiscing about a vacation we'd taken years before to the beautiful, mystical Pu'uhonua O Hōnaunau ("Place of Refuge") National Historical Park in Hawai'i. Ancient warriors and others who came to this spiritual sanctuary (if they survived the harrowing swim in the treacherous bay) were granted refuge in this island paradise.

Then it hit me: it's vital to seek places of refuge on the healing journey, even if at home.

Where's your place of refuge?

- Perhaps it's a special room or sacred space in your home or in nature. Even a bathtub soak is a refuge.

- Consider interior places of your mind accessed by meditation, visualization, vision quests, or daydreams (more on this in future chapters).

- Write about your place of refuge in your journal, sketch, paint, or collage it. The more energy you pour into it, the more alive it becomes and the easier it is to travel there in your mind when you need to.

In addition to the place of refuge in your mind, you can create a serene healing sanctuary in your everyday world. In the Scandinavian culture of my ancestors, the word *hygge* (pronounced *hyoo-guh*) is defined as "a quality of coziness and comfortable conviviality that engenders a feeling of contentment or well-being."[30] Creating a peaceful healing sanctuary of *hygge* needn't be expensive, time-consuming, or energy draining. It's as simple as creating space in your home (or bedroom, or even a bit of space on a nightstand) and amping up the healing vibe.

If you have an abundance of money and time, by all means, knock yourself out. But you can accomplish this by simply rearranging what you already have. That's what I did. The point is, do what you can do within your ability and budget to create a welcoming, nourishing space for rest and healing.

Within a month of being flat-on-my-back bedridden, my husband helped me transform our bedroom into a healing sanctuary. On my nightstand is a Himalayan salt lamp, several crystals, a Tibetan singing bowl, and Palo Santo essential oil mist.

The dresser has several get-well cards containing inspiring messages from friends and family and a vase of flowers from my husband. A wee plastic dragon reminds me to be fierce about robust self-care and self-advocating. We hung a small bunch of dried lavender from my mother's garden and moved light-catching crystals from our sunny kitchen to our bedroom window overlooking our forest's towering pines, cedars, and blue sky.

We relocated a small corner bookshelf from my office studio so my beloved books are close at hand. As a practical matter, we moved a small, pretty Florentine table beside the bed that serves as a place for my laptop, phone, journal, etc.

On a far table are treasured talismans representing the four elements: a smooth stone from a Scottish loch, a raven feather, a fig candle, and a seashell from a Caribbean island. These simple treasures from times spent in nature are reminders of the healing power of Mother Earth.

- **A Sidebar about Talismans**—Joseph Campbell tells us, "The reluctant hero requires supernatural forces to urge him on, while the willing adventurer gathers amulets (magical items) and advice from the protector as aid for the journey."[31] In addition to adorning your abode with talismans, we can carry these items—charged with our intentions for protection or healing—as something to reach for in trying times. Much like an athlete with "lucky socks," I wear a black tee-shirt bearing a vintage Asian dragon as a talisman and reminder to be robust with self-care, breathe the fire of passion for life, soar when possible, and be fiercely authentic in speaking my truth.

Also on the talisman table lives an Apple HomePod, gifted to me by my stepdaughter, that is often playing healing music: sounds of ocean waves, rain, crystal bowls, and Reiki or meditation music. Music elicits a vibrational shift of mood and outlook in an instant. Use it to your advantage.

The bedroom colors were already perfect for healing and rest—the calming twilight shades of lavender, periwinkle, indigo, and burgundy.

This is my happy place for healing where I can rest, recover, and hibernate. The whole setup made convalescing a bit more tolerable by holding sacred space for healing.

There came a point when my physical capabilities expanded. My place of refuge extended too. As I began spending a couple of hours a day up and around the house, I became more work-fluid: working from bed, on the deck amongst cedars and pines, by the garden, from the kitchen as morning sunlight streamed in, or by the wood-burning stove on cold winter days. It helped make work more in alignment with healing.

What would your healing sanctuary look and feel like? What makes you comfortable? Safe? Calm? As you curate your space, think of all your senses: music, colors, special treasures, plants, scents, talismans, art objects, the elements, as well as practical necessities. Fill your sanctuary with pictures of people you love, photographs of places you've been, team pennants if you're a sports fan.

Create a Shrine to Healing

It all started when I was down for the count in December 2016 with the ruptured disc. Near the end of one day, I assembled the elements of a little shrine on our bedroom dresser. It reminded me of my intention for healing with a fir-balsam candle, a large amethyst crystal, statues of Quan Yin (a reminder to practice compassion) and Ganesh (remover of obstacles), and a diffuser for essential oils.

This wasn't my first shrine. For decades we've had little altars around our house—one for creativity in my studio, another in Ken's office, one in the garden, one to honor departed loved ones for *Día de Los Muertos*.

For centuries, people the world over have made personal shrines—indoors and out—as a visual and energetic reminder. They can be a nod to nature (feathers, seashells, crystals, leaves, flowers), spirit animals, ancestors, angels, Jesus, Buddha, St. Francis, Our Lady of Guadalupe, or favorite goddesses. The point is for it to be meaningful to you, a place to offer blessings, prayers, intentions, and gratitude.

Consider making a shrine to your own healing journey in a manner that reflects your personal beliefs and elements of your mindfulness ritual. Keep it energized often with the following practices:

- lighting candles, incense, or fragrant herbs (sage, palo santo, sweetgrass, mugwort)
- offering your prayer, intention, blessing, gratitude, or wish written on a piece of paper
- adding a fresh flower, leaf, acorn, seashell, shard of beach glass, crystal, river rock, feather, or other offering

Create Meaningful Daily Rituals

Rituals connect body and spirit, focus the mind, and hold sacred space for prayers, intentions, and gratitude. Rituals signal crossing the threshold of our inner worlds.

Robin Wall Kimmerer, remembering family camping trips and her father's coffee ritual, tells us a ritual "marries the mundane to the sacred. The water turns to wine, the coffee to a prayer. The material and the spiritual mingle like grounds mingled with humus, transformed like steam rising from a mug into the morning mist."[32]

I was into ceremony and ritual long before the devastating disc rupture. They have a way of bringing such simple magic, awareness, wonder, and intention into every day. When I healed enough to finally be able to move about and do some things for myself, I revisited ways to incorporate daily rituals back into my life. They are essential to my healing.

Here are some favorite rituals that make my life more grounded, sacred, and enchanting:

- Upon awakening, I follow the thread of my dreams and jot them down in my dream journal.

- Before my feet hit the floor, I give thanks for being alive, for my health, and for all the blessings in my life.

- The act of brewing tea or coffee is a ritual too when I bring mindful awareness to the task. I bless it, intentionally sip, and graciously accept this blessing from Mother Earth, reminding myself to step into the flow and ride it like water.

- My refreshing shower or relaxing bath is a ritual for finding clarity and cleansing my spirit as well as my body.

- On sunny days, light rays illuminate the crystals in my window at just the right angle (forty to forty-two degrees, to be precise) to paint rainbows around my room. I take a mindful deep breath, admire their beauty, and enjoy this illuminated moment.

- In the breeze, melodic wind chimes in the tree outside my window are a harmonious reminder of mindfulness. I gift myself a moment just to breathe. In fact, throughout the day, I program my breath as a blessing. For example, breathing the word *peace* or *love*.

- Every day I burn a candle, incense, palo santo, or sage. It's an opportunity to get centered and send healing thoughts of love and light to friends, family, and all sentient beings.

- Being aware of beauty and mindful of inspiration raises vibration. Visualization, meditation, affirmations, intentions, prayer, ringing Tibetan or crystal singing bowls, singing, humming, and chanting also raises vibration, and hence, healing.

- I aim to live by the seasons, in rhythm with the moon and tides, and sync my rituals with them.[33]

11
YES, PLEASE!

> Look for the helpers. You'll always
> find people who are helping.
>
> —Nancy Rogers (mother of Fred Rogers)

You cannot make this long healing journey alone. In addition to your medical team, you'll need a support network of friends and family helpers.

I wasn't particularly good at asking for help, but I had little choice when the most debilitating disc rupture occurred and left me flat on my back, unable to do much of anything for myself. The silver lining was, of course, an opportunity to learn to say "yes, please" and allow others to help.

Friends made soup, bought groceries, ran errands, and sat by my bedside to keep me company. One friend drove me to appointments in distant cities to see neurosurgeons and doctors. Another spent hours pulling weeds and planting flowers in my garden so when I was able to sit outside there'd be beauty to feed my soul.

I'm surrounded by the love of many good friends who helped me through this journey. Friendship is strong medicine—the cure not found in any pill.

> The ones who show up when you haven't
> even asked but exactly when you need them,
> are this life's most beautiful gems.
> —Stacie Martin

Who's on Your Team?

Your team isn't only the people who happen to be around. You'll want to learn who has what skills and whom you can count on for specific tasks.

For instance, you'll need errand-runners, worker bees, domestic helpers, and those among whom you can rest and recharge. You'll want teachers, wayfinders, and healers, for sure. Sometimes you simply need someone to bear witness and hold space, to listen when you've hit a rough patch or setback, to offer a hug when you're in tears, or to send prayers.

Be open to what gifts and skills the people in your life can bring and know that most people *enjoy* helping. Loved ones may feel helpless in being unable to fix your health crisis. You can help them find a way to do something meaningful.

Asking for Help

For nurturing women and strong men accustomed to taking care of things or being of service to others, it can be difficult to accept and graciously receive help. But we must. Accepting help is an act of self-compassion, not selfishness—a sign of strength, not weakness.

Moreover, the more challenging the health crisis, the harder it can be to figure out what you need. The following will help you break things down.

Know Your Limitations and Where You Need Assistance
Think of it this way: *Where will you spend your precious limited energy?* Be honest with yourself about what you can and cannot do. Simplistic as it sounds, make a list of all the daily activi-

ties you can no longer do, tasks large and small: housekeeping, cooking, going to market or pharmacy, walking the dog, driving anywhere. Prioritize the list.

Identify Your Tribe
Start with your inner circle and treasured kindred spirits. If you don't have a spouse, parent, child(ren), or grandchild(ren) in your inner circle, then expand the circle of helpers: ask friends, extended family, neighbors, colleagues, community members, your church/temple, or club members who can help. Identify those who will accompany you on this journey and be your all-important support network. *Who's on your team?*

Ask For Help
Speak your truth. Ask your tribe to take your hand on this journey by helping with specific tasks. Give them options from your list. Speaking our needs prevents us from feeling things are completely out of control. Hire someone if you must. Accept help in all its forms. If you're helping someone who's ill, one of the best questions you can ask is "How can I best support you?" Similarly, if you're the person in need of assistance, make your needs known: "The best way you can be there for me is ____."

Say Yes
Every minute spent taking care of your health will pay dividends to your recovery. Accept that you need assistance now. Just say "yes, please!" and "thank you!" Let others help in ways that tax your own health.

Graciously Receive with a Grateful Heart
When people help—whether it's to carry your bag of groceries to the car, cook you a nice dinner, or loan you a walker—remember to express sincere thanks. It's more than an utterance of the words. Deeply feel appreciation. It's soul-soothing.

KATHY HARMON-LUBER

> They may forget what you said
> —but they will never forget how you made them feel.
> —Carl W. Buehner

PART 4

YOUR SELF-DIRECTED HEALING JOURNEY

We should not feel embarrassed by our difficulties, only by our failure to grow anything beautiful from them.

—Alain de Botton

12

COMPASS INTUITION: LEARNING TO LISTEN

> If prayer is you talking to God,
> then intuition is God talking to you.
>
> --Dr. Wayne Dyer

Humans have two types of intelligence: one type is in our minds, of course, but we also have our intuition. Intuition is the way we know things, sense things, without thinking them through logically—the knowledge comes from someplace deep within. It's the place inside you that connects with Source, God, Creator, Spirit, the Universe, angels, or whatever you prefer to name it. Intuition is our compass and navigation system: the gut instinct, hunch, gentle nudge, whisper, tug of the heart, voice of the soul, Inner Healer. Call it what you will, everyone has intuition. When you practice listening for it and to it by trusting and following its lead, its wisdom will help you heal.

In the animal world, intuition, or instinct, is a primary means of perception. Today, many cultures worldwide rely upon intuition for survival. Western culture, not so much, and I believe we're the worse for it. Your healing crisis is a crucial time to cultivate and tune into your intuition. Everything you need for the healing journey is within you. When we allow our intuition to flourish, we become walking antennae picking up energy and attuning to synchronicity.

When a healing crisis occurs, it's human nature to look outward for answers (doctors and other medical professionals, healers, gurus, etc.). In addition to legitimate health professionals, there are snake oil salesmen and scammers of all stripes trying to get rich off the fears and desperation of the ailing. Profit-driven pharmaceutical companies and social influencers aim to motivate us to buy stuff. Contradictory guidance abounds. External energies and pressures like these can drown out the voice of our Inner Healer.

If we don't listen to our instincts, we may become confused and disoriented at a time when we're most vulnerable. Intuition helps with wayfinding when we're lost or blazing a new path on the healing journey.

How Does Intuition Speak?

> Albert Einstein called the intuitive or metaphoric mind a sacred gift. He added that the rational mind was a faithful servant. It is paradoxical that in the context of modern life, we have begun to worship the servant and defile the divine.
> —Bob Samples, *The Metaphoric Mind*

How many times have you said "I should have listened to my instincts," or "Why didn't I trust gut?" or "I didn't follow my heart"? Perhaps you ignored a sign or synchronicity. Been there, done that, right?

When you look inward, quiet the noise, and listen, your Inner Healer speaks wisdom. For example, the day before my disc rupture, I had returned from a two-day business trip to onboard a new client. Prior to the trip, I was already experiencing severe back pain. Every instinct said *don't go!* Oh, I heard my intuition, all right. I just didn't heed it. I *wanted* to go and ignored my Inner Healer. It was the "last straw" for the bulging disc, which led to the rupture. Might the disc have ruptured anyway? I'll never know. You can be sure I won't disregard my intuition again.

Here's an intuition story with a happy ending. Shortly after COVID-19 lockdowns in 2020, I began having massive heart palpitations late at night—terrifying galloping horses stomped around in my chest for hours on end. I was sleep-deprived and scared, which made matters worse, of course. Until then, I'd never had any issue with my heart.

I had a hunch it could be a combination of anxiety and my anti-inflammatory and nerve pain medications. After describing my symptoms and my hunch to my doctor, I was surprised when he said, "I've noticed your instincts are always spot on." They were this time too. The biggest reminder was my doctor's parting words, "Follow your gut." It's all the encouragement I needed to continue heeding my intuition.

No one knows your body better than *you* do. Your body and soul are your best teachers. Their voice is your intuition, your Inner Healer, your compass pointed at true north. You are the healer and hero you've been waiting for!

Intuition Is a Muscle

Freedom of speech is a basic right we passionately ensure for others—yet sometimes we deny it to our own inner voice. If your intuition is wearing a muzzle, it's probably gone silent. If your intuition is weak or you don't hear its voice at all, no worries. The good news is intuition can be developed, like building muscle or learning a fun new game.

> The quieter you become, the more you are able to hear.
> —Rumi

It requires stillness, quiet, and athletic listening (i.e., full attention and deep listening) to hear the wise voice inside:

- Learn to recognize your Inner Healer's soft whisper of what feels right (or wrong), and listen deeply. *How do you "hear" it? Where in your body do you feel it? Your gut? Heart?*

- Be observant of external synchronicities and signs.

- Pay attention to hunches, tugs on your heartstrings, and clenches in your gut.

- Engage in dialogue with your inner voice, asking for healing wisdom (be patient, as there's not always an immediate answer).

- Follow its lead by (responsibly) heeding its guidance.

- As you observe its wisdom and how it serves you, develop trust.

- Keep a journal to help witness the wisdom of your intuitive hunches, noting how you followed through.

Whether you hear intuitive rumblings now and again or whether you're completely disconnected, you can do this. It's there right now, simply waiting for you to tap in. Start where you are. You wouldn't set out to learn a dance step or new sport by trying it only once and determining you can't do it, right? If you're already a pro at trusting your intuition, congratulations—keep on developing it. It will serve you well.

Once you're in the flow of intuition, it's beautiful and life-changing.

If a door opens and your instinct says it's right, "leap and the net will appear," as John Burroughs famously said. Pay no mind to those unreasonable, squabbling fears.

The Intuitive Healing Approach

One of my teachers, Puma Fredy Quispe Singona, says, "Listen to yourself first and last." I'd add that you should listen to your medical team along the way, weigh their advice, be your own advocate, and ultimately follow your intuition. *What resonates in your heart (or gut)?*

There was a time when humans remembered how to heal through the old ways of the grandmothers, ways based on intuition. Now each of us needs to return to listening to our intuition.

This means *trust yourself.* Don't give your power away—not to doctors, caregivers, family, or friends. Trust you will know (or interpret) what healing modalities in your Toolkit resonate with you. Sometimes when we're in the company of others—even those we love—it's difficult to hear our own small voice crying out for self-care. Make some alone time to deeply listen to your inner voice.

Some well-meaning people have given me bad health advice over the years. It was contrary to my own instincts, but occasionally I followed it, and I've never said, "I'm glad I ignored my gut and tried that." I've learned the lesson: *Follow your inner guidance.*

Taking this a step further, trust your inner wisdom to interpret your ailment's relevance at this point in your life. Now there's something to contemplate!

The intuitive approach to healing is holistic—seeing the whole person. It doesn't look only at vital signs or the broken leg or the one diagnosis as most Western doctors do. Seek out functional medicine and naturopathic doctors who will work with your intuition.

When you have a chronic illness or debilitating injury, out of pure necessity you must become your own nurse or physician's assistant: monitoring setbacks, progress, and flare-ups; doing copious research from reputable online resources, books, and health professionals; and then following your instincts about what might work for you.

Doctors will tell you that what works for one person doesn't necessarily work for another. There's only one *you* in the entire universe. Only you can know what makes sense for *you*. Fully inhabit your intuition, your instincts, and your likes/dislikes. Listen to everyone—of course—do your research, discern what feels right to you, and walk that path.

Intuition is your superpower, your own unique flavor of magic. Follow it and the magic happens. Follow it to your healing. You need it now more than ever.

Deeper Dive Exercise

If you've spent your life trying to stifle your intuition, finding it can be a bit like an archeological dig. Intuition is a developed skill. As with any skill, it's honed and made stronger by daily practice. This can be fun![34]

- First, unplug from your devices (like sensory deprivation, it awakens your Inner Healer). Banish the to-do list. Go someplace quiet and safe where you can be alone with your thoughts: a favorite spot in nature, a special room in your house, your backyard, or a balcony.

- Be still. Just breathe for a bit. Enjoy being in this present moment. Pay attention to how you feel and what catches your mind's attention.

- The more you work with your intuition, the clearer and more reliable it becomes. Ask, *What would help me feel better, physically (or emotionally), right now? What's ailing me today? What emotion am I feeling? Do I really need to go out later and do X or would rest better serve me? Do I need a nap? Exercise? Protein?* Do you hear a whisper?

- Hold space for the bigger questions: *What do I need to know in order to heal? What interests are calling me?*

What would I like to learn? What would make me happier? What do I truly want for the rest of my life? What is my illness/injury's relevance in my life's path?

- Listen. *What pulls you? What speaks?*
- Write down your observations and any intuitive messages.
- Practice this daily and throughout your day when possible. Then you'll be ready when you're faced with making the big decisions: *How do I feel about the risk of this surgery or that medication?*
- Meander, following the thread of your curiosity. It's how we find treasures hidden deep inside us. Remember Tolkien's words: "Not all those who wander are lost."
- Then grab your courage, dive deep, and *follow* your inner compass.

It's called trusting your intuition. It's where the magic begins. It's where you discover . . .

> The real voyage of discovery consists not in seeking new landscapes, but in having new eyes.
> —Marcel Proust

Authenticity

> Know thyself.
> —Inscription on the Temple of Apollo at Delphi, Greece

Michael Meade tells us, "The most common reason for despair and alienation comes from not being who we are at the core of the soul."[35] Intuition is the voice of the soul. When we don't listen to it, we aren't being our authentic selves or remaining true to our soul's calling.

The problem is, society minimizes authenticity. Often our parents and relatives, teachers, friends, partners, workmates, and bosses try to mold us into what they want. It's your duty to yourself to unlearn this, to dig deep and find your authentic self and be unapologetically *you*.

It's important to realize we cut off our intuition when we don't practice acceptance of our authentic selves, and our hearts close down as a result. But, like water from a faucet, intuition *can* flow again.

> At any moment, you have a choice, that either leads you closer to your spirit or further away from it.
> —Thich Nhat Hanh

In addition to being an essential tool for healing, intuition can help you find and navigate your authentic way forward in life. When you know what lights you up with passion, you'll know your authentic self. Intuition points the way.

Joan Walsh Anglund famously said, "A bird does not sing because it has an answer, it sings because it has a song." Your song is your passion, purpose, and dreams.

What song does your heart long to sing?

> Let yourself be silently drawn by the strange pull of what you really love. It will not lead you astray.
> —Rumi

That which you are seeking is seeking you. If you keep hearing a message or getting a sense or feeling, it's something in your soul calling you. As long as it's ethical and harms no one, know it's right for you. Follow it. It will lead you deeper into your authentic self.

Intuition is your compass pointing toward your own true north. There is power and seduction in *yes*. Say yes to the voice of your intuition and see what doors open up for you.

> Whatever you think or feel, the universe says yes.
> —Robert Moss, *Sidewalk Oracles*

There's not another person in the universe created the way you are. You have a gift—no one in the universe has your unique expression. You are 100 percent unique. Your power—including your healing power—lies in your uniqueness. Be the real, authentic, badass *you*. Own it. That's where you'll thrive. Goethe tells us, "As soon as you trust yourself, you will know how to live."[36]

When Intuition Says No!

> If you don't know how to say 'no' when you need to,
> your body will say it for you in the form of illness.
> —Dr. Gabor Maté

Hives, nausea, fatigue, headaches, pain, panic attacks, mental imbalance, burnout, nervous breakdown . . . these are a few of the ways our bodies say no to what is not best serving our health—or worse, damaging it. It's a wake-up call: our intuition is instructing us to pay attention, do things differently, radically simplify, or just say no.

For most of us, it takes some time to understand our body's way of getting our attention, doesn't it? This was a long, difficult lesson for me—repeated several times, as it must be for some of us slow learners. Each time I didn't heed my intuition, my body's signals of *no!* cranked up in volume and intensity. Until I listened.

> There is deep wisdom within our very flesh,
> if we can only come to our senses and feel it.
> —Elizabeth A. Behnke

Not heeding your intuition by saying no to an activity or person who's not in alignment with your health and happiness comes with an exorbitant cost.

How much do you want what you want? Is it worth a health setback?

Ask your Inner Healer for guidance when considering an activity or work project:

- What's the cost to my physical, mental, and emotional well-being? What negative impact?
- What's the toll on my energy currency?
- Does it detrimentally cut into self-care time?
- Will it require recovery time?
- On balance, is it worth it?

What's the cost of going out with friends when you're feeling really bad physically? Or saying yes to an ambitious work project although you're overwhelmed with fatigue?

What's the price of saying yes? If it will negatively impact your health and require much recovery time, it's seldom worth the price. Just say no! Admittedly, this is a huge challenge in the "just do it" era. But sometimes, say no we must.

This goes for emotional health as well. Scientific research has proven the link between negative emotions or a traumatic event and the onset of sickness.[37] We must pay attention to our inner world and process our emotions before they cause illness. Get qualified professional help if you need talk therapy (help to process intense negative emotions and/or depression).

Listen to your body moment by moment to solve issues of pain and frustration and process them before they explode into an unhealthy reaction that triggers health decline.

That is one piece of the puzzle. Another is setting good boundaries (by saying no when intuition advises it) to keep suffering at bay. Setting boundaries is not selfish—it's self-positive self-preservation.

Let's get you started on creating some health-positive boundaries. Consult your intuition in the following ways:

- How does your body say no? What symptoms does your body send you to signal no?

- What situation(s) or activity(ies) might be triggering this symptom? In other words, what are you doing in your life that might not be in the best alignment, no longer serve you, or go beyond your body's physical/mental bandwidth?

- What can you do about it? What boundaries can you create? Can you easily stop the activity? Cut that person out of your life? Scale back the duration or frequency of the culprit? Not take it personally?

- How can you radically simplify your life to better support your health? What can you say no to in order to create more space for better self-care? Simplify your life to find greater meaning. Peel away everything nonessential.

- Do you need help in better processing negative emotions so as not to trigger illness or flare-up episodes in the future?

This exercise is especially vital if you find yourself caring for others: children, grandchildren, aging parents, your business or co-workers, friends, and/or your community.

This is the beginning of healing because it means you're on the way to identifying habits that may have led you where you are today. Defining better boundaries and listening to your Inner Healer—intuition—will help you get to the next level of healing.

> We do not become healers. We came as healers. We are.
> Some of us are still catching up to what we are.
> —Clarissa Pinkola Estes

13

FIGHT FOR IT: ROBUST SELF-CARE

> There are days I drop words of comfort on myself
> like falling leaves and remember that it is enough
> to be taken care of by myself.
>
> —Brian Andreas

We must fight for our health—of body, mind, and spirit—and our dreams.

When it comes to health, most people don't realize that where they are right now in their lives is a culmination of all their choices, all the decisions they did and didn't make about self-care. By making positive self-care choices, we can create a healthier life with greater well-being.

In the year leading up to the disastrous disc rupture, I knew I should have been practicing better self-care. Yet I was so busy with life, I was convinced I didn't have a choice. There wasn't time to fit in the self-care my body needed. I was working ten-to-fourteen–hour days and serving on three boards of community charities. In my spare time, I made art and photography, performed classical flute on weekends, and traveled. I also swam three or more hours each week, walked daily, and went to the gym. On top of that, my husband and I spent a glorious (but painful) vacation in coastal Oregon and a holiday by the sea in Carpinteria.

I intuitively knew I needed robust self-care. Truly, I hadn't made any semblance of self-care a priority. I paid dearly for that choice.

What Is Robust Self-Care?

Self-care springs from the river of self-love and compassion. Be kind to yourself. *Do you treat yourself like a precious treasured object, or do you treat yourself (or talk to yourself) as you'd treat no other human ever? Your child? Your pet?*

Robust self-care is more than good grooming and sleep hygiene:

- Eat foods free of toxins that wreak havoc on your compromised, fragile body: organic fresh foods, non-GMO foods, wild-caught seafood, and free-range/grass-fed protein sources without antibiotics. Read labels like a super sleuth and purchase the highest quality food you can afford.

- Select personal care products with pure, natural ingredients and avoid those laden with poisons such as sodium laureth sulfate (found in shampoos, bubble baths, moisturizers), aluminum (in deodorants, it's linked to breast cancer), and formaldehyde, toluene, and dibutyl phthalate (toxins found in nail polish). Those are but a few common toxins. Do your research and make purchasing decisions accordingly.

- Do more of the things that improve your condition (see Chapter 16, "Super Sleuthy You").

- Do none of the things that worsen your ailment. Use good judgment and common sense. Don't attempt to do tasks beyond your bandwidth that might injure you or cause further decline. Remember it takes a long time to heal, so avoid further injury and setbacks in the first place. The key is to be mindful (stop multitasking).

- Take care of your mental/emotional balance through quiet time for reflection and contemplation, creative pursuits, meditation/mindful awareness practices (download a bell of mindfulness app), and living in the moment.

- Practice relaxation daily to recuperate your health, restore well-being, and recover your balance. Medical researchers have found that short bursts of relaxation/rest, even ten minutes long, combat the damage of stress and restore balance to our bodies and minds.[38]

- Forgive people who've hurt you. It doesn't mean what they did was okay, but you've accepted they're human and you're ready to move on with your life without the baggage of emotional attachment. Forgiveness is a powerful healer.

- Follow your passion, what lights you up. This is the ultimate form of self-care! If something drains you, it's not sustainable. Give yourself permission to do what energizes you. *What lights you up today?* Do what fills the tank and reduce what drains the tank. Ask, *What do I need right now to feel good?*

- Be your own fierce protector and warrior woman / warrior man. Nurture yourself with dogged tenacity. Keep showing up for yourself again and again. Some days it helps to visualize putting on a coat of armor, war paint, warrior or ninja garb, or bodhisattva stance—whatever it takes to fight for the care your fragile, vulnerable self needs. You are so worth it.

Self-care doesn't mean selfishness, though some friends, family members, and society in general would want us to believe otherwise. We're no good for anyone else if we aren't at our best. Only you know how to get yourself there.

A New Carrot

When we're deep into the healing journey, self-care should be our number one priority. With external pressures, we often allow our health to be hacked[39] by our technology, work responsibilities, family obligations, social commitments, and misplaced concern about what others might think.

What's keeping you from making self-care your top priority? Do you think tending your health is just another obligation on the to-do list, or do you do it with love? Think about all the things you tend in life and how much time you spend doing them. How does that amount of time compare to tending to your own self-care?

Self-care takes time. In some cases, it takes financial resources. Self-care might require you to miss activities you'd rather pursue. Self-care might make you unpopular in your social circle. When we think about the "cost" of self-care—in time, money, fear of missing out, and so forth—we must shift our focus and define the new "carrot." By this I mean pivoting to *I'm going to feel much better in a couple of minutes/hours/days if I do [insert self-care here] now/daily/forever.*

With the inoperable ruptured disc, I made a conscious all-in choice of radical self-care—resting, taking care of my spine, giving up everything that caused pain and further damage, and finding inner peace. Any other choice would have demonstrated a lack of self-compassion and self-love.

Have you seen those signs in car windows that say "Baby on Board" or "Precious Cargo on Board"? Yep, that's you. Treat yourself like a precious object, like a newborn, because you're just as vulnerable on your healing journey. Be gentle with yourself. Show self-compassion. *Would you treat a helpless child the way you sometimes treat yourself? Would you treat your worst enemy the way you sometimes treat yourself?* I realize this might be hard to accept, especially if you're a man or a strong woman who has always taken care of others.

But we must make a life-long habit of treating ourselves with kindness, gentleness, unconditional love, compassion, and acceptance of our vulnerabilities. Just as we would a newborn or our pet.

Honor your body—your soul's temple—by treating it like a treasure.

Because it is.

Do the Important Things First

When we're down for the count, we're forced to pay attention. If we develop mindfulness, tune in, and become deeply aware, we'll hear our bodies telling us what they really need in order to heal.

We push ourselves hard and harder to do more and accomplish more on less and less sleep and unhealthy meals, filling our lives with busyness—and precious little of the most important things.

I taped this reminder to my bathroom mirror: *Do the important stuff first.* For me, it's taking robust care of 1) my health and well-being and 2) my relationships (family, friends, colleagues, community, world). Let me ask you this: *What's your important stuff?*

The COVID-19 pandemic brought this sharply into focus for many of us. As people began dying around us, we realized *life is short.* Some of us shifted, beginning each day by doing the most important things first.

If you're on the healing journey, place self-care first and foremost in your day, every day. Robust self-care requires:

- unconditional self-love and compassion
- time (yes, we must make time for self-care)
- laser focus

- course correction when needed (like recovery days after you overextend yourself)
- unwavering commitment to fight for your self-care

When you do those things, you'll improve your condition. Isn't that what you ultimately want? Do the important things first:

I am intentional about how I spend my irreplaceable time today.
I do the most important things first.
Today, robust self-care comes first.

As your navigator on your healing journey, I'm giving you a Self-Care Permission Slip (get yours at <u>SufferingtoThriving.com</u>).

When to Begin?

If you're just now realizing you've not been practicing good self-care (for months, years, or a lifetime), don't beat yourself up. Start where you are. Start today.

I know this isn't easy. I still struggle with it too. It means I hit the reset button again and again. And that's okay.

Arrange space and time in your life for daily self-care. Remember how good it feels. Engrave this feeling in your mind. Make it a treat to look forward to.

In recent years, there were long stretches of time when self-care occupied the majority of my day. Today it's far less. There's no one-size-fits-all. Give your body what it needs when you need it, as much time as it takes.

Sean Patrick Flanery put it another way: "Do something today that your future self will thank you for."

> If you have been chosen for a particular and challenging task,
> face it with heart, courage and wit,
> and never lose sight of your compassion.
> —Noble Smith, *The Wisdom of the Shire*

14

TAKING INVENTORY: ABILITY, NOT DISABILITY

Do what you can, with what you've got, where you are.

—Squire Bill Widener

Here is one of my journal entries, written one year after my disc rupture:

> *I haven't done art, photography, or music for over a year now. I cannot physically pick up my camera or flute without severe pain. I cannot stand at an easel or sit in a chair, which makes the messy work of painting in bed out of the question. I feel like my life ran off without me. I'm a shell of the person I was. I am beyond exasperated . . . and depressed. . . . It's as though pieces of my heart and soul are missing. Journaling helps, but it will never replace music, or the joy of creating a painting, or the thrill of that moment of magic in the camera. I need to figure out a new way.*

Writing those words took me down a new path. Sure I could have chosen angry, bitter frustration. I actually tried that for a few days but decided I didn't want to live my life that way.

Instead I chose to figure out what I *could* do. I kept thinking back to years before when I was executive director of a Los Angeles agency that assisted people with developmental disabilities and helped them focus on *ability*, not *disability*, to achieve their full potential.

Aha, an interesting twist of fate. I reminded myself to focus on my own abilities rather than inabilities. I contemplated, *How can I create a new life for myself and maximize my abilities? It's clear now's the time to stretch and grow.*

It was exciting! I got curious—*With these health limitations, what* can *I do? What do I want to do? What's my new dream?*

When one door closes, another opens. Suddenly, I was looking for all the opening doors.

It was a mindset shift: from disability to ability, from limitation to the gift. Hope is finding the things you love and loving them in perhaps a new and different way.

> We must be willing to get rid of the life we've planned,
> so as to have the life that is waiting for us.
> —Joseph Campbell

Taking Inventory

I first needed to face what I could no longer do, starting with everyday activities. Lying flat on my back in bed, I grabbed paper and pen and got to it. The list was long and depressing: unable to get into the shower, drive a car, walk, swim laps, dance, etc.

Then I populated the list with my passions, things that bring me joy. For example, I couldn't play classical flute. I went from performing professionally nearly every week to nothing, overnight. I couldn't—and still can't—sit at my piano keyboard for ten minutes. As mentioned, I couldn't paint at an easel or hold a camera.

I took a deep breath and simply accepted that, for now, I must let those things go. Hopefully not forever.

Next I thought, *What* can *I do?* In another column, I wrote "What am I capable of doing, still preserving my current ability, without risk of setbacks?" Sometimes, that's all you can do. Sometimes, that's enough.

ADAPTATIONS

Then I researched what work-arounds would enable me to have a better quality of life. Adaptations enabled me to stay as active as possible from bed while keeping pain from ramping up:

- I cannot sit at my office desk to work (even with adaptive spinal cutout and lumbar cushions), so I purchased a portable desk from which I can work comfortably. The game-changer is an Avana orthopedic bed pillow support system.

- For driving, I wear a medical-grade back brace and use a spinal cutout seat cushion plus lumbar support.

- A cane or walker enabled me to walk without falling. This was difficult at first. The problem, of course, was my ego—the cane made me feel like an old lady. Until I fell. From that moment forward, I used the cane and accepted it. It enables me to walk safely for ten minutes. It's a far cry from the five-plus hours a week I walked prior to the rupture, but boy, am I grateful for every step I can take today. Freedom!

What adaptation will help you to be safer? More comfortable? More active? Do what you must.

Here's another game-changer. Fifteen or more years ago, basic activities continued to cause spinal discs to bulge or tear, resulting in enormous pain and long recovery periods. I saw yet another orthopedic surgeon, one of many, who wouldn't operate: it would entail a fourteen-hour surgery, low odds of making pain and mobility any better, and a risk of paralysis.

Exasperated, I pleaded for anything that would help me figure out what I could safely do, avoiding activities that might cause my spine to collapse. He referred me to a physiatrist who improved my life immensely. I didn't even know what a physiatrist was (a physical medicine and rehabilitation physician who focuses treatment on function and on the whole person in their real-life environment). This little-known type of doctor can help you relearn everything so you have more ability and, importantly, don't reinjure yourself. Physiatrists are skilled at helping us find adaptations aimed at making us more active and comfortable.

This physiatrist literally taught me how to sit, brush my teeth, get into/out of a car, get in/out of bed, stand to cook meals, take a shower, use a cane/walker, and so on—all the basic life activities we take for granted, yet, if done incorrectly for our conditions, may actually cause harm. She encouraged me to use a medical-grade lumbar traction machine, a ball chair at my office desk, and a back brace. All of these adaptations gave me more ability.

Importantly, she helped me see what I need to say no to in order to preserve my fragile, collapsing spine. For example, I was no longer permitted to do any housework (this did not break my heart). I was crushed to learn my favorite pastimes, walking and hiking, were now considered high-impact activities. Likewise, no gardening. No biking. The gym? No way. *Never lift more than five pounds.*

I protested! "I must do the housekeeping—we can't afford a housekeeper." Her reply was, "You can't afford not to." So we rearranged our lives to accommodate my spine with the end goal of halting deterioration.

What Can You Do?

Today, decades after doctors told me I'd be in a wheelchair, I'm grateful to say I am not. It all worked: I have less inability and more ability. In some strange way, after being forced to lie horizontally in bed, I've come alive in unexpected ways: my writing (daily journal, this book, chapbook of poetry, my day job) has replaced flute, painting, and photography. My written creativity has become finetuned, a source of great joy, and I've blossomed (even winning an international poetry contest and having poems published in poetry journals).

Years ago, a little summer bird outside my bedroom window was singing, trilling louder, more excitedly, and more passionately than all the others. I wondered, *Perhaps it's a young bird singing its first song? Maybe it experienced the thrill of flying for the first time? What would make* me *so thrilled? So passionate?*

Music helps us to live from our heart center. *How could I make music my medicine?* When I could no longer dance every day, I realized I could choreograph dance in my mind (which I still do when I hear great music). I rediscovered my Native American and Celtic flutes, frame drums, singing, and guitar.

When I could no longer hold my camera, I realized I could put it on a tripod and stand for five minutes to photograph. It's how I created my photography portfolio *Dream Blossoms: Dreams Blossom*—and the cover of this book—five minutes at a time, punctuated by long hours recovering. But still, I did it! It's fulfilling, in a very different way, of course, but fulfilling nonetheless. Do I miss playing my flute, splashing paints around, and traveling? Definitely. But I now realize that for everything lost something is gained. For now, this is enough.

Here's my inventory list, as an example of what you could try:

What I can't do:	*What I can do instead:*
Classical flute, keyboard	Sing, Native American flutes, Irish whistle, drums, guitar
Ride horses	Sketch horses (and more!)
Garden	Photograph flowers, put plants on my windowsill, admire nature
Dance	Choreograph dances in my mind

Perform flute gigs	Listen to music, meditate, enjoy sound therapy
Go to concerts and shows, travel	Watch films, take virtual classes, read books, call friends
Walk, swim, hike, bike	Do physical therapy, write poetry, publish this book, deepen my studies in the healing arts

I've found joy in unexpected places. You can too.

Your Turn

We must bloom where we're planted. Right now, you're firmly planted on the healing journey. Use this time to bloom into something new. Now's the time—not some far-off day when you're "all better." "Someday" is today.

Nothing more than this moment is assured. Now is the right time to reframe your disability into a new set of abilities and possibilities. You might aspire to be a rose, but today, you're a sunflower. Bloom true, and love yourself for being the best sunflower you can be. Turn your face toward the sun of new possibilities.

It's time to transform your inabilities into abilities. So what exactly *can* you do? Let's assess your "new normal" by making two inventory lists:

1) Recognize what you can no longer do.

2) For each activity, identify at least one thing you *can* do, focusing on new and different opportunities. Hopefully you'll discover something fun, positive, and/or rewarding. *Have you always wanted to learn a new language? Take up a hobby? Explore a hidden talent? Catch up on films?* You get the idea.

What's your list?

I can no longer _____.	Instead, I can enjoy _____.
I'm unable to _____ right now.	Until I'm able to do this again, I can have fun with _____.
I cannot _____.	This adaptation might make it possible: _____.

Fill this list with activities, passions, interests, adaptations—get creative with possibilities.

Never give up on trying to find ways to overcome your inabilities to accommodate your passions. Think about it: Employers are required to make *reasonable accommodations* for their employees' disabilities. Yet I've encountered people who are physically compromised and don't attempt to find their *own* reasonable accommodations. Don't let that be you. Never give up on yourself, your dreams, or your life.

Power and manifestation flow to where your attention goes. Keep your attention trained on ability, not inability. Change your perspective. Explore something new. This is what you have control over (and precious little else).

If you can discover and cultivate these resources, they'll serve you well for the rest of your life.

> Experience is not what happens to a man;
> it is what a man does with what happens to him.
> —Aldous Huxley

15

MAXIMIZE YOUR MEDICAL APPOINTMENT

> Chance favors the prepared mind.
>
> —Louis Pasteur

As with any fulfilling journey of discovery, it's important to get organized first. Before we know the best route forward, we'll need to understand exactly where we are now.

To get the most out of this book, consult your medical team to get answers to the questions below. Western medicine excels at diagnosis, so be sure to avail yourself of it and learn the following:

- What's my diagnosis?
- Do I have the best doctor for the condition?
- What's the prognosis?
- What will improve the prognosis?
- What can I do to make the condition more manageable?

- What makes it worse? (Because it's critically important to preserve what we've got, especially with chronic and/or progressive conditions.)

- Talk to others who have your condition: What have they learned? What worked for them? What didn't? Which doctor(s) do they recommend?

If you don't have answers yet, no worries. Let's look at ways you can start to get answers by getting the most out of consulting with your medical team.

Every medical professional will have opinions about what you should do, but they don't inhabit your body and mind. So you'll need to be a tenacious advocate for yourself, as you'd be if you were advocating for a child. Because, truly, your sick or injured self is a lot like a wounded child who needs a strong, empowered advocate. You'll begin by learning to trust your intuition, as we discussed previously. Then you need to make sure you're taking full advantage of any medical appointments you have.

Consider the average length of a doctor visit is just 17.4 minutes.[40] According to a 2018 study, most US physicians (around 65 percent) spend somewhere between 13 and 24 minutes with patients. About one quarter spend fewer than 12 minutes, while roughly 10 percent spend more than 25 minutes.[41] You may have waited months for this appointment only to have a few minutes with the doctor. It's easy to get distracted by a diagnosis or recommendation and forget to ask your questions or not paint a full picture of your circumstances in a brief visit.

How can you make the most of it? Like most things in life, it helps to be prepared. A week before your appointment, write a one-page summary to share with your doctor. Bulleted points make it easy for your doctor to read questions, concerns, and relevant medical history.

Include the following elements in your summary:

- Reason for the visit (e.g., new condition or follow-up appointment)
- Current symptoms (are they constant, aggravated by triggers, eased by rest or activity?)
- Medications you're taking, as well as vitamins, supplements, over-the-counter products, and any complementary treatments (acupuncture, massage, meditation, naturopathy, homeopathy, yoga, etc.)
- A brief medical history, past medications tried, and if relevant, MRIs/X-rays/CT scans, blood test results, diagnostics, and a list of other doctors, chiropractors, or other medical professionals seen (for first-time visit)
- A brief "day in the life" of how your condition affects/limits your work, sleep, hobbies, family/other relationships (at the appointment, we usually look our best and stretch even to get to his/her office, sit in a chair, and look like we've got it all together)
- Your questions (if you don't know what to ask, look online for recommendations[42])

Remember, there are no stupid questions. The right question could save your life or dramatically improve your health, so don't be reticent.

In addition to the preliminary questions above, here are some of my go-to questions:

- What can I do to improve the condition?
- What triggers should I avoid so as not to make things worse?
- What complementary medicine options are there in addition to Western medicine?

- For difficult diagnoses or risky procedures, ask, "If I were your child or spouse, what would you advise?"

It's essential to get your summary to your doctor prior to your visit so they have time to digest it and consider a course of treatment before they see you. If your doctor accepts patient emails or has a patient portal online, submit it there. Ask the receptionist when you make the appointment how best to deliver this. If your doctor is old-school, you'll need to bring a printout. Ask the assistant to ensure the doctor reviews it prior to seeing you.

At the appointment, be sure the doctor addresses all your questions. (Bring your own copy of your summary to refer to.) Be certain you understand their answers fully. You're probably not a doctor—it's okay not to know stuff. Ask for clarification of anything you don't understand. Don't be shy about asking *more* questions in order to understand your condition, prognosis, and treatment options. You have control of determining what's right for you. Write down answers and recommendations. If possible, take someone with you. Two sets of ears are helpful in this situation.

If your doctor says they cannot help you (which has happened to me), be sure to ask, "Whom do you recommend?" or "What type of specialist(s) should I see?" I saw numerous orthopedic surgeons before one said as a last resort, "Perhaps you should see our physiatrist." I suffered from debilitating spinal conditions for twenty-five years before learning what a physiatrist does.

Recordkeeping

It's important to keep good records, especially if you have a long-term chronic and/or progressive condition. It will serve you well if you change doctors and need to provide a medical history or if you decide to apply for disability.

You could keep a notebook with section dividers for MRIs/X-rays/CT scans, blood tests/diagnostics, medications currently/previously taken, doctors' visit notes, and a list of doctors seen (including outcomes). One friend keeps an additional notebook of her *daily* medication dosages, pain level, amount/type of exercise, and other activities she's able to do. It's a good way to track progress and easily see if something is improving—or impeding—your progress. It's especially useful when you're trying new supplements or alternative treatments.

Do You Have the Right Doctor?

As you know from life, who we hitch our stars to profoundly influences the trajectory of our lives—for better or worse. It's true for your medical team, too, so it's critically important to identify the most credentialed, successful doctor(s) you can afford.

Shop for a doctor as you'd shop for a new house or car. They must be the right fit for you. You might need to consult with two, three, or four doctors to find one who fits the following description:

- has the right expertise and successful experience in treating your particular condition (is it their specialty?)
- listens, answers your questions, and is caring and compassionate
- views you holistically
- is affiliated with a highly ranked hospital (in case you need it)
- is up to speed on best practices and latest breakthroughs
- is open to integrating Western medicine and complementary, functional, regenerative, and/or naturopathic medicine practices

- has a strong success rate (In other words, what percentage of patients have improved with surgery? Have any died as a result of following a protocol? Based on your situation, what results would they expect for you? What's the likelihood of success? The higher the risk of the prognosis, surgery, procedure, or protocol, the more vitally important it is to conduct your due diligence. Your best possible health—or your life—could be at stake.[43])

In some cases, you might need to curate a medical team. For example, a GP, rheumatologist, physical therapist, pain management doctor, physiatrist, and surgeon. It helps enormously if they're already a well-oiled collaborative team, but that's not always possible. The point is, build a team that maximally addresses all your needs and doesn't rely on only one person should an urgent situation arise.

Medical Trauma

> One's dignity may be assaulted, vandalized,
> and cruelly mocked, but it can never be
> taken away unless it is surrendered.
> —Martin Luther King, Jr.

The sad truth is our doctors can hurt us while we're in a vulnerable state. Today I'm fortunate to have an excellent, caring medical team and good health insurance that enables me to see the best doctors, but I didn't always. I've been through many doctors who didn't listen and were dismissive, condescending, and devoid of compassion. Then there are doctors with a terrible bedside manner, those who appear to listen but don't really hear you, and those who think the problem is all in your head.

These types of encounters only add more trauma to already relentlessly horrible experiences.

Do you have a medical trauma story? You're not alone. Remember, there are many excellent, compassionate doctors out there. If you experience an incident of medical trauma, find a new doctor.

> I can be changed by what happens to me.
> But I refuse to be reduced by it.
> —Maya Angelou

16

SUPER SLEUTHY YOU

*The important thing is not to stop questioning.
Curiosity has its own reason for existing.*

—Albert Einstein

We're all desperately trying to find answers to questions: *What will heal me? What will relieve the pain? How can I prevent a flare-up? How can I live a more 'normal' life, despite my ailment?*

Healing knowledge is not a secret, however—it's been around for thousands of years. With the internet, we have ready access to information about both traditional healing modalities and miracles of modern medicine.

But let's face it, we don't know what we don't know. When I embarked on this healing journey in earnest, I quickly realized I had a lot to learn. People constantly recommended I pursue some therapy, treatment, or supplement. I tried many of them, casting about for something that worked, but I didn't do it haphazardly. I investigated, experimented, and tracked my progress.

Healing yourself—or at least having the best possible life with your condition—requires you to find your own path. Because we're all unique, one size doesn't fit all. Do your due diligence and tailor the most supportive protocol best suited to your health challenges.

In advocating for your health, it's not enough to have a great medical team and someone like me as your guide. You're the hero you've been waiting for.

You must become a super sleuth. This can be fun! Let's get curious.

The first step is to understand what you're working with: the name of your condition, what makes it better/worse, and what's the next step. Western doctors will get you this far. But here's what most people don't realize:

1) There's so much more help out there, and if you do your research to identify complementary modalities, they might work for you.

2) Every incremental improvement can contribute to less discomfort, more energy, better sleep, stronger immunity, greater mobility, fewer flare-ups, etc.

Without the miracle of modern medicine, I'd probably have died in childhood or been crippled by now. I have great respect for Western medicine, especially its diagnostic capabilities. Accept the best Western medicine can offer, but realize integration with complementary medicine protocols can accelerate healing.

The National Institute of Health's National Center for Complementary and Alternative Medicine (NCCAM) classifies complementary and alternative medicine therapies into five categories or domains:

1. Alternative medical systems
2. Mind–body interventions
3. Biologically-based treatments (herbalism)

4. Manipulative and body-based methods (e.g., chiropractic and massage therapy)
5. Energy therapies[44]

Complementary medicine is more popular than you might imagine. According to a nationwide survey, Americans spent $30.2 billion out-of-pocket on complementary health approaches.[45]

My Western-trained doctors gave me dire predictions that my health conditions would progressively worsen. In taking a holistic, integrative approach, however, my healing has been exponential.

Here again, you must be your own best advocate—asking questions, doing the research, following clues, being systematic in trying new avenues. The rewards can be great.

Let's get super sleuthy.

Where to Begin?

- Start with firsthand experience. If you have a common condition, ask people in your network or community to share what works for them (or didn't). If your condition is rare, find a reputable online community. Some medical societies and research organizations[46] have chat rooms where you can post questions for a doctor. Always check with your own doctor before trying something new.

- With a few clicks, you can access a treasure trove of information on the internet. Again, it's best to stick with reliable sources[47] that can help you not only understand your diagnosis but also what makes it better or worse, symptoms to watch for, standard and complementary protocols, when to see your doctor, questions to ask, etc.

- Look up prescription medications[48] to understand possible side effects and interaction warnings.

- Search these topics by your condition (for example, "vitamins and minerals for X condition"):
    - complementary and functional medicine
    - naturopathy
    - epigenetics
    - homeopathy
    - Ayurvedic medicine
    - food sensitivities/allergies
    - acupuncture/acupressure
    - reflexology
    - benefits of yoga and meditation
    - vibrational medicine
    - Reiki
    - magnet therapy
    - infrared and cold laser treatments
    - chiropractic procedures
    - myofascial release massage
    - traction
    - heat/ice treatment
    - anti-inflammatory diet[49] (similarly, lectin-free diet, heart-smart diet, Mediterranean diet, histamine-free diet, etc.)
    - herbal and flower tinctures
    - dream healing

Many of these holistic treatments have been practiced for thousands of years in Chinese medicine, Indian Ayurvedic healing, and other healing practices around the globe.

- If your condition is physically structural, research adaptations that might help for sitting, walking, reclining, driving / being a passenger in the car, and other daily life activities. (See Chapter 14, "Taking Inventory," for more.) Explore every option and determine what will help you be mobile and safe.

- Read books, listen to credible podcasts, watch videos, and see what resonates. Your body knows what makes sense if you get quiet, listen to your Inner Healer, and keep an open mind.

- Follow every lead on the trail and take good notes of findings and new leads to explore. While there's useful information to be found online, as we know, dubious information and snake oil salesmen are rampant. Your health is precious, so always take the utmost care to verify reputable sources.

- Once you have a list of things you'd like to explore, ask your medical team if it's advisable and safe to pursue. My doctors encourage complementary medicine, however, once I mentioned supplements to explore and they advised against because of interaction with medications or the inappropriateness of certain procedures. Consulting with your medical team first will save time, money, and possibly your life.

Try Something New

Perhaps certain foods are making your health issues worse or an activity or habit is making your condition more painful. Perhaps acupuncture or Chinese herbal supplements would improve your ailment. Armed with options from your sleuthing—and your doctor's approval—the only way to know for certain what works for you is to be systematic.

It's a simple process. Pick one thing to try and give it time to determine if it makes a noticeable improvement. Otherwise, if you try too many things at once, your results will be muddled and inconclusive. For instance, you begin trying five new things in the same week. Next week, you notice an improvement. Something worked! But what was it? You don't know.

Early on I made the mistake of starting a new CBD formulation and turmeric brand (both pricey) at the same time—it worked! In a couple of weeks, the new regimen had taken the edge off my pain. But which treatment worked? Or did they work synergistically? I didn't know. I eliminated them both for a couple of weeks and then started over again, introducing one at a time. Turns out only one had a significant impact. This little experiment saved cash in the long run.

If you're physically injured, employ a similar method when starting a new exercise. Otherwise, if you add ten new exercises and wake up the next day with severe inflammation, you won't know whether you overdid it that day or if it was one exercise in particular.

Food Sleuthing

The same sleuthing process I've outlined for treatments also works for food and supplements. In sixteen years, my rheumatologist never mentioned the connection between autoimmune disease progression and foods/supplements.[50] Almost everything beneficial I've learned about detrimental foods, beneficial supplements, and the anti-inflammatory diet has been through my own research and seeking advice from naturopaths and doctors with a complementary medicine focus.

These discoveries changed my life. In fact, with food choices and supplements alone, my asthma and osteoarthritis have disappeared and autoimmune progression has plateaued (doctors said it would progressively worsen).

Let's take a deeper dive into food sensitivities. Nightshades, gluten, sugar, lectin, dairy, caffeine, alcohol, sodas, processed foods, and additives like MSG can cause bodily reactions like inflammation, swollen joints, fatigue, tummy troubles, hives, asthma, anaphylactic shock, and autoimmune flare-ups. Food sensitivity can be a silent killer. It was in my case. When my GP ran tests and I eliminated several sensitivity issues more than a decade ago, I recovered my health.

Everyone's body is different. Some people are fine with gluten. For others, it triggers inflammation. Ditto for sugar. Lectins (e.g., peppers, lentils, peas, soybeans, cashews, quinoa) and nightshades (eggplants, tomatoes, potatoes, etc.) are especially interesting, as these plants secrete toxins to protect their seeds from being eaten by animals. Get this—most animals avoid lectins and nightshades because they recognize their toxins! We humans eat these seemingly healthy foods without realizing they're actually making us feel bad.[51]

How to Find Food Sensitivities

First, pick your culprit. What food(s) do you intuitively feel might be causing an issue? Let's say refined sugar because it causes issues for nearly everyone. In fact, a recent study showed that cutting 20 percent of sugar from packaged foods and 40 percent from beverages could prevent 2.4 million cardiovascular disease events, 490,000 cardiovascular events, and over 700,000 cases of diabetes in the US.[52]

For one month, cut sugar out of your diet completely. Replace it with organic honey or stevia. Read every label carefully for this hidden culprit. In a notebook or calendar, record when you begin this experiment and then daily observations about any changes in your health. *Are you feeling less pain and swelling? How's your tummy feel? Energy levels? Mood swings?*

After a month, gradually re-introduce sugar into your diet for a day or two. *How's that working for you? Do you notice a difference in how you feel? Worse, perhaps?*

Once you've established sugar is bad for your health, then you can begin cutting out another suspect. Remember, it's important to test only one thing at a time. If you test two simultaneously and have a reaction, you'll not know which is problematic. Keep going until you feel you've identified all your problem foods. A little research on anti-inflammatory and/or low-histamine diets will give you the list of the most common culprits.

Once you know your triggers, make a list of foods to avoid. Put it on your refrigerator. Take it to the grocery store. I've learned I can keep my autoimmune issues from spiraling out of control—and beat them into remission—by avoiding my triggers. This means I don't eat pasta, pizza, bread, coffee, croissants, licorice tea, sugar, or (perhaps the most difficult of all) my beloved tomatoes, potatoes, peppers, and eggplants—nightshades, all. I've been avoiding some of these foods for decades, so when I do a rare splurge, I pay for it.

What motivates you more: avoiding misery or indulging in the fleeting pleasure of a food that hurts your body? When you're ready to avoid unnecessary suffering at all costs, it's easy to avoid the triggers. Your long-term health is worth it! Do I miss eating pasta, eggplant, tomatoes, and bread? Oh yeah. Am I healthier without them? Without question, yes! It's totally worth it.

I admit, for the first month it's difficult. But then you find your sweet spot:

- fewer swollen, inflamed, stiff joints
- diminished pain
- fewer flare-ups
- less gastric distress
- better energy, mental clarity, and overall health

When your pain and suffering become bad enough, you'll try anything, and when it works, it's easy to make it a lifestyle habit.

The flipside of this is to explore superfoods with proven wellness benefits, like mushrooms (e.g., reishi, cordyceps, chaga, shiitake), dark leafy greens, berries, green tea, etc. *What superfoods will you explore?*

All or Nothing?

What if you cannot cut a trigger food out of your life completely? Remember, all progress is incremental. Let's say you normally eat sugar every day. If you can't go cold turkey, try cutting back by 50 percent. Cut back from two cookies to one, from a whole granola bar to just half. Or eat sugar every other day. Once you've tried this for a week, cut back by 50 percent again for the following week. Continue to wean yourself from it until it's gone completely.

It sounds almost unbelievable that food can change your health, but there's a lot of research behind this. I've given the topic so much real estate in this book because it's been transformational to my health. I've always been a healthy eater; cutting out the food sensitivities was the game changer.

The choices you make in every moment shape the trajectory of your suffering and your healing. You choose between pain or pasta . . . suffering or sugar . . . agony or coffee. *Do you want to feed the misery or avoid it?*

Do one more thing that makes you feel better. Then another. Treat it as a game—a scavenger hunt!—whatever motivates you.

Is It Worth It?

This sounds like a lot of work, I know. But consider this: in 1986, I was diagnosed with Raynaud's Disease (in the autoimmune family of illnesses). At that time, it was just a name as I had no symptoms except my hands and feet would turn cold and white in Washington, DC's cold weather. Fast forward to winter 2006: I was deathly ill, battling gangrene, close to losing a couple of toes, nearly unable to get to work, and looking ten years older than my age. I felt like death warmed over. I called in sick a lot, and colleagues asked if I was going to be okay.

Today I feel better than ever—and look younger and healthier than I did then—which I owe to being a super sleuth when it comes to avoiding flare-up triggers and diligently taking beneficial supplements. While it hasn't cured this incurable, progressively worsening disease, I've stemmed—even slightly reversed—its progression, which doctors said couldn't be done.

But I haven't stopped sleuthing. I recently stumbled upon a study about the link between forty-one autoimmune diseases and childhood trauma.[53] Doctors never mentioned this. I discovered it by being super sleuthy. This underscores the importance of being an empowered advocate for your own health.

It benefits you to learn how Big Agra's processed, genetically modified, pesticide-laden foods correlate to disease—which Big Pharma tries to fix with more drugs. Many medical professionals (certainly not all) are in Big Pharma's pocket. In the words of a pharmaceutical executive: "We're in the business of shareholder profit not helping the sick."[54]

What we eat impacts our health. If you haven't already, you'll find it's health-transformative to adopt a clean (no processed foods), organic (no pesticides), non-GMO (genetically modified organism), mostly plant-based diet (eat the rainbow). If you eat meat, purchase grass-fed, free-range, antibiotic-free meat/poultry, and wild-caught seafood.

A little knowledge can be an amazing thing when it comes to the arc of our healing journey. In case you're curious about my time-tested successful protocol, here's a snapshot.

- Avoid trigger foods.
- Adopt the anti-inflammatory diet.
- Build a healthy gut. (When you optimize gut flora, you heal the inflammation at the root of much disease and pain, and you'll recover your health. I've done this. It works!)
- Reduce stress through meditation.
- Aim for eight or more hours of sleep every night.
- Utilize physical therapy exercises, traction, TENS unit, heat, ice, myofascial release, and massage.

- Benefit from acupuncture/acupressure, magnet therapy, vibrational energy, and sound healing.

- Explore functional medicine, naturopathy, Ayurvedic medicine, regenerative medicine, homeopathy, and so on.

- Learn all you can about the mind–body connection.

For decades, my doctors have not only encouraged me to explore complementary modalities but often recommend new approaches to try. But what if your doctor dismisses complementary medicine? Get a second opinion from a doctor of osteopathy, doctor of functional medicine, doctor of naturopathic medicine, or doctor of regenerative medicine. These fully licensed doctors take a whole-person approach and can help you with personalized nutritional (or other) interventions.

I'll leave you with this reminder I have posted on my bathroom mirror: *Be open to changing how you live your life every day.*

Once you've discovered what changes work for you, it's all about sticking with them.

17

STICK-WITH-IT-NESS

> Perseverance is failing nineteen times
> and succeeding the twentieth.
>
> —Unknown

Health impediments don't go away with reading a book but by actually trying different modalities and then integrating successful ones into your life.

Most people who experience a meteoric rise to fame in any field—becoming "overnight" sensations—will tell you it took countless hours of consistently practicing their craft to achieve mastery. All progress is incremental: step by step, mile by mile. It's true whether you're building muscle, losing weight, raising children, creating a career, designing a house, mastering an instrument, growing a garden or forest, or learning tennis.

The same holds true for the healing journey. You can't try something for a day, or even a week or two, and expect life-changing results. Commit to six months. Be disciplined—it's how systemic change is made. As with any change we seek, healing is incremental.

Essential to incremental progress is stick-with-it-ness. Decide to make positive changes, then consistently and tenaciously stick with them until they become good habits: normal, ritual, even unconscious. It takes an average of 66 days for a new behavior to become automatic.[55]

Commit to perseverance, as if preparing for a voyage to uncharted territory, because this is indeed uncharted territory to a new way of being.

STEP BY STEP TO YOUR NEW LIFE

As you aim to improve your health and life, what habits are worth investing your time in? Grab your list of actions from the last chapter. Rank it in priority order with the biggest impact actions/foods/supplements topping the list. *How can you make that a habit? What do you need? Where will you find the time in every day to do it?* Note it in your calendar every day for two months. Then stick with it. That's how I used supplements to transform my health, built strength through physical therapy, and developed a meditation practice—by sticking with it every day.

Here's an example. Decades ago, the highly respected Dr. Cynthia Watson (internationally known for blending Eastern and Western medicine with great outcomes) helped me heal from chronic bronchitis and sinus infections. She warned me before beginning the protocol—echinacea, goldenseal, astragalus, ginger, high dosages of vitamins B and C (including IV drips), etc.—that the vitamins and supplements had to be taken consistently for at least six months.

When we're suffering miserably and urgently wish to heal, we may want a right-now fix. Good health is a long game, however. If you might have your pain for the rest of your life, then taking six months to try something to reduce it is probably worth it. I've stuck with it all these years and have seen a life-changing impact over decades. Had I not given Dr. Watson's protocol the prescribed amount of time to prove its effectiveness, I'd still be miserable. I've had similar success dramatically improving asthma, osteoarthritis, and autoimmune disorders.

The key to sticking with it is to make it a practice. According to author Fenton Johnson, "A habit is a way of living that you follow because it's what you did yesterday and the day before and the day before that. A practice is a way of living that you create and renew every day. A habit is a way of being that controls you. A practice is a way of being that you control—a deliberate (ad)venture into the unknown."[56] It is intentional.

Not Working?

Try everything that makes sense to you and your medical team. Even in "failures," we learn. It's not a linear journey. If one path isn't working after a while, try a different path. Come from the perspective of failing your way to success. Remember what Edison said? In the midst of developing a new invention, someone asked him, "Isn't it a shame that with the tremendous amount of work you have done you haven't been able to get any results?" Edison smiled and replied, "Results! Why, man, I have gotten a lot of results! I know several thousand things that won't work." Edison stuck with it through failures to success.

Every moment presents the opportunity to try again.

Small setbacks can obliterate our calm and perseverance—but only if we let them. Keep moving forward and trying new things with a calm heart and mind and stick-with-it-ness.

Start now.

When traveling, I enjoy visiting gardens—especially those with ancient trees. They remind me of people who ask, "When is the best time to plant a tree?" The age-old answer? "The best time is twenty years ago, but the second-best time is today."

Begin today. If you have a practice of inner work, it will get you through this challenge. In a month or so, you'll be astonished by how your life has changed in the most remarkable ways. In six to twelve months, you'll be transformed.

18

BEARS DO IT, BEES DO IT

> Doing those deeply unfashionable things—
> slowing down, letting your spare time expand,
> getting enough sleep, resting—is
> a radical act now, but it is essential.
>
> —Katherine May, *Wintering*

We can't expect to heal by continuing to live our lives full throttle and popping meds. To maintain our health, sleep, rest, hibernation, slowing down, and getting quiet are essential. We can learn this vital lesson from the animal kingdom. We're familiar with bears' hibernation, but did you know honeybees sleep five to eight hours a day?[57] Whether observing our domesticated cats and dogs or looking further afield to ailing animals in nature, it's evident they innately know self-care:

- prioritize sleep
- rest often
- hibernate when you need to
- slow down

- get quiet

The benefits of these five essential self-care practices are tremendous. They can help you heal optimally and will strengthen your resilience.

Cultural Pressures Work against Self-Care

> Go slowly, breathe, and smile.
> —Thich Nhat Hanh

Everything in today's overstimulated world is racing fast. Society has little patience with anything that isn't immediate. *Take a pill. Get the surgery. Have a speedy recovery.* No time to rest and sleep. No time for robust self-care. If we're ailing and exerting ourselves at breakneck speed out there in the world, it's at the expense of our recovery, long-term health, and well-being.

Societal pressures keep us hamsters on a wheel. Despite research showing that taking time off from work improves efficiency, "41% of employees reported feeling like they were being 'vacation shamed' . . . being made to feel a sense of shame or guilt by coworkers, their supervisor or their employer for taking time off to go on vacation."[58]

Several years ago, a friend reflected in an email, "It's this 'responsibility' ethic/belief that keeps interfering with me being okay taking the time necessary for me to heal. Maybe that's one reason why I create *dis-ease* to justify my need to retreat from the world." That's something to ponder.

For the sake of our health, we need to empower ourselves to take the time necessary for rest.

This has been a hard lesson for me. In January 2017, a month after the disastrous disc rupture, I wrote this:

> *As I looked back over my journal from ten years ago, I was shocked to discover I'd written about a bulging disc that sent me straight to bed "to slow down, rest, heal." Perhaps the bulging*

disc happens in order for me to slow down, rest, heal . . . I need to change the way I care for myself so this doesn't continue to happen. I urgently need rest.

We experience so much noise, busyness, and deadlines in today's world. We need to be practicing robust self-care, prioritizing sleep, taking "rest stops," hibernating for healing, slowing down the pace, and getting quiet. Health setbacks give us the opportunity to take stock and find a new, wiser way forward.

Sweet Sleep

Sleep is strong medicine. As young, strong, healthy people, we probably didn't realize this bit of wisdom. But when stricken with an ailment, it becomes a profound truth and as vital as the air we breathe. During sleep, elegant repair work happens in both body and mind.

Sleep scientists tell us, "Sleep is one of the most important things we do. . . . Not getting enough sleep is linked to an increase in the incidence of many conditions, including cancer, autoimmune disorders, cardiovascular disease, and Alzheimer's."[59] And that's not all. One study found that "people who did not sleep well react more emotionally to stressful events the next day and do not find much joy in positive things."[60]

Unfortunately, health setbacks can rob us of the sleep our bodies vitally need, as in the case of painsomnia (or fatigue so extreme that sleep is elusive).

How to Optimize Your Sleep

- Structure your life to accommodate as much sleep as your body requires for recuperation. Ditch the alarm and let your body dictate how much you need. If it's a fourteen-hour sleep marathon, so be it.

- Eat a light evening meal at least four hours before bedtime with no snacking afterward.

- Avoid alcohol and stimulants, replacing them with naturally decaffeinated herbal teas (avoiding mesh bags which release microparticles of plastic into your body) like chamomile, valerian, passionflower, mugwort, other relaxing tisanes, or golden milk.[61]

- It sounds obvious, but be sure to take your vitamins in the morning. An exception to this is magnesium, a sleep aid.

- Unplug from your devices and dim ambient light in your bedroom a couple of hours before bedtime. When you're ready to turn in, ensure your bedroom is completely dark. Remove electronic devices from your room or store them at least three feet away for optimal sleep.

- Live in rhythm with nature and the seasons by turning in earlier in winter when nights are long and a little later in summer.

- Dab a few drops of organic nutmeg, lavender, or vanilla essential oil (diluted in a carrier oil) on your wrists—or in a diffuser—before lights-out.

- Practice breathing exercises for relaxation, meditate, visualize, mentally review your gratitude for the day, and/or explore yoga nidra. If anxiety or fear consume you, try the Cone of Protection visualization in Chapter 36, "The Guided Journey," to create a safe space.

- If you're easily wakened by slight noises, play white noise—like the ocean or gentle rain—throughout the night.[62]

Try the steps above and see how better sleep can improve your health. Getting more sleep helped me begin making quantum leaps in healing.

Get Your Rest

At some point in convalescence, we're told to rest. Few of us are good at it, but rest we must if we're serious about healing.

In addition to a good night's sleep, health returns in the "rests," the moments between things. Think about it: the rests between musical notes give music its structure. We hear and appreciate music *because* of the rests. We can enjoy better health when activity is offset with rest.

As every elite athlete knows—little breaks recharge. What's more, after an especially intense training or performance day (or whenever their bodies signal it), athletes recognize they need a "rest" day.

It's essential we tend to our own health as we'd look after a sick loved one. You'd give them the rest they needed, right? Tend to your own rest in the same spirit.

It's challenging to put "rest" into practice. When my rupture first happened, I was totally bedridden and had no choice. I couldn't do anything but sleep and rest. The challenge arose when I finally was able to get out of bed for a couple of hours a day. As life accelerated, rest became more of a mystery. *How much rest do I need? When do I need it?*

For decades, I'd lived life full-on. Lots of exercise, travel, play. Hard work, little rest. My motto was "rest when you're dead." In learning to rest, I've realized there's no one-size-fits-all. Trust your intuition on when and how much to rest and what activities make you feel rested (or not).

When it's impossible to carve out large blocks of time for rest, slowing down at intervals throughout the day helps. Many years ago, I began a practice that improved my ability to work in a more balanced, rest-fueled way. But like many good habits, one day it slipped by the wayside.

So I reinstated this habit for times when there's no time for rest. It goes like this: every hour I take five minutes or so to turn off all the noise, get quiet in my mind, close my eyes, and just breathe deep healing breaths. After that mini-break, I return to work sharper and sometimes with a new perspective or creative idea. (Another way to accomplish this is to use a bell of mindfulness app.) If a breathing break isn't your thing, try an awareness meditation or daydream.

These "rest stops" between work, family obligations, and other responsibilities are where our bodies and minds reset. We become more relaxed, balanced, and grounded when we rest. Try it for a week, listen, and get to know yourself. *What does my body want me to know? What is my ailment trying to tell me? When I rest, do I have less pain? More energy? Better immune response? More clarity of mind? Sharper focus? Stronger body?* Make this a practice, and you'll change your life and health in amazing ways.

Hibernate

In an especially rough patch three years into my disc healing process, my GP emailed me: "The more I ponder, I don't believe it's in your best interest to just keep upping the doses of meds. We know what it is that's initiating the flare-ups, and that is what has to be addressed . . . please slow down the work. Rest should indeed help, but not a day here and there . . . at least a week or two."

This happened at the onset of the COVID-19 pandemic. As many people were losing their jobs, my work increased rather significantly. There were financial pressures: my husband, a teacher, was unemployed most of that year. I didn't have time to rest.

Deadline stress is a trigger for my autoimmune flare-ups, excruciating nerve pain, and—for the first time in my life—daily heart palpitations that lasted three terrifying months. I urgently needed to keep working, but my body was screaming for rest. So I followed my doctor's orders and for a couple of weeks, I hibernated from it all.

Hibernation is where we try, like a bear in winter, to step away from the world and into our healing sanctuary for an extended, undisturbed period of time for self-care. It sounds difficult, but like everything on this healing journey, the rewards far outweigh the inconveniences. Hibernation is a reset, and with it, my health improved.

Slow Down and Get Quiet

Healing can't be rushed. There's no quick fix. Healing isn't so much a problem to be solved as a process to go through. Yes, it's a journey. Take it slow.

Healing takes . . . well, as long as it takes. Accept it. Ride it out, floating in the middle of the river. Trust. Allow. Don't fight it. Loosen your grip on control. Be agile. Manage expectations. For most humans, myself included, this is not easy. But it's not impossible either. Busyness is a choice. Slowing down for self-care and healing is also a choice.

Practice coasting. I don't mean shirking responsibilities at work or with family duties (although if your condition is quite serious, perhaps you must). Rather, don't push yourself or strive to do things *beyond your current health capacity*. Disrupting the stress response by slowing down is essential.

Remember, our bodies know how to heal if only we give ourselves time to rest, recharge, recover, and recuperate. When we get quiet and rest, we come into our own healing power. Being sick or injured can leave us feeling weak. Weakness is not powerlessness. Ignoring self-care is powerlessness—you're giving away your power to heal.

Slow your pace. Find a new rhythm. When learning a new piece of music, we musicians slow down the pace. *Why not slow your life pace to learn how to recuperate?*

Honor this time for healing with sleep, rest stops, hibernation, slowing down, and getting quiet.

PART 5

THE THRIVING SPIRIT

I am a divine creator.

—Joe Dispenza, "What the Bleep Do We Know?"

19

KEYS TO PEACE: ACCEPTANCE, SURRENDER, AND LETTING GO

> Peace is the result of retraining your mind to process life as it is, rather than as you think it should be.
>
> —Dr. Wayne Dyer

Healing doesn't come from outside you—although it's easy to believe you should search for it there. Yes, look externally for remedies and adaptations, but not only there. Healing is an introspective journey. Like peace and happiness, healing is an inside job. Most doctors agree—attitude is everything. A large factor in experiencing fulfilling healing is in your head, which means you have more control over your progress than you may realize. Isn't that empowering?

One day I chatted over tea with my friend and Reiki teacher about my health crisis and how the lessons of acceptance, surrender, and letting go are like an onion. We peel away one layer to find the next layer and the next. She calls this The Advanced Practice journey. It's not easy, but it's key to releasing suffering and finding peace.

With some diagnoses, there are good prognoses, promising procedures/surgeries, or innovative miracle meds. But what happens when we see no way out? No promise of improvement, only decline? Then what? There's no going back to life as it was. *It is what it is*. To find peace, we must accept this.

> Whatever the present moment contains,
> accept it as if you had chosen it.
> —Eckhart Tolle, *The Power of Now*

Benefits of Choosing Acceptance

> This place where you are right now
> God circled on a map for you.
> —Hafiz

When you first get the scary diagnosis, you might experience shock, disbelief, and denial, and then you ask "Why me?" But if you take to heart the message in Chapter 1, "Everybody Hurts," the question becomes "Why not me?" All of life is imperfect, and you'll be more content if you can embrace *wabi-sabi*[63]— *life's imperfections and messiness.*

> There is no perfection, only beautiful versions of brokenness.
> —Shannon L. Alder

You did nothing to deserve this health crisis. It wasn't part of your life plan, but face it, this is where you are today, and it sucks. *It is what it is*, and to find peace within, you must accept it as best you can. It's certainly easier to rage, blame, or pity. When you're ill or hurt, the hardest thing to do every day is to accept *what is*.

Don't beat yourself up. You're doing the best you can under challenging circumstances. Your body is working very hard to heal. Accept that this is where you're at now on your life's path and that everything will resolve at the right time.

Accepting things for what they are is extraordinarily powerful. Acceptance

- builds resilience (our ability to bounce back from life's challenges)
- minimizes mental and emotional suffering
- enables us to embrace our authentic selves
- brings inner peace and harmony
- comes before deep healing and transformation

The secret to not suffering is accepting "This is my new life. This is who I am now. These are my limitations." Sometimes it's about accepting "I am not okay." Choosing to accept pain, fatigue, malaise, brain fog, immobilization, or something worse as your constant companion doesn't mean you won't strive to improve. Acceptance means turning to face the truth of your circumstances—again and again, day after day—not struggling against it.

Acceptance is about loving the life you have at this moment, warts and all. Not pining for the good old days or living in the future. Not ignoring your circumstance or distracting yourself with multitasking, devices, drugs, or alcohol.

When I stopped resisting and accepted my situation, it was liberating. Acceptance, along with its pals surrender and letting go, will transform your life.

Longanimity

I learned this new word: *longanimity*—a disposition to bear injuries patiently.[64] How does one become *longanimous*? I'm sure acceptance is at the threshold. What's needed is to cultivate a habit of being okay with *what is*.

During the COVID-19 pandemic, everyone's life was disrupted. Family and friends died, folks lost their jobs, domestic violence and child abuse increased, people became homeless, and businesses were lost. This is suffering on an epic scale, no doubt about it. But some people experienced a different kind of suffering—self-imposed—stemming from the perceived inconvenience of wearing a mask, quarantining, social distancing, and the disruption of their "normal."

But if we practice longanimity, then that kind of suffering doesn't put down roots and grow wild.

Like you, I wrestle with the acceptance of things small and large—including radical unknowingness with no expectation things will be okay again. I must remember Maharishi Mahesh Yogi's words: "If something bad happens, it doesn't matter. If something good happens, it doesn't matter." Life happens. By removing expectations about the outcome, we don't get upset when things go wrong, so the energy doesn't get stuck. It flows—the optimal condition from which to live your life of peace, happiness, and healing.

With acceptance, you'll grow. Without acceptance, you might become bitter. Let's choose the good stuff.

> Heaven on Earth is a choice you must make,
> not a place you must find.
> —Dr. Wayne Dyer

Accept how your healing journey has been necessary for growth and transformation. Take time to honor what needs acceptance, then surrender and let go of what no longer serves you. That's how we get into the flow of life.

> Flow with whatever may happen and let your mind be free.
> Stay centered by accepting whatever you are doing.
> This is the ultimate.
> —Zhuangzi

Surrender

Once you've accepted your circumstances, surrender is a vital step for getting into the flow and birthing a new life from your health crisis.

Surrender doesn't mean giving up. Not at all. It means *trust life*. Stop struggling. Surrender to what is becoming. John O'Donohue wrote, "We live between the act of awakening and the act of surrender. We live between morning awakening, and bedtime surrender to sleep. Between birth and death. Between the lives we had and the little 'death' of that life. Between awakening to the purpose of your healing journey and surrendering to it. The common thread of all these examples is, finding Beauty there."[65]

To surrender is to open space in your heart, body, mind, and day-to-day life for a new way of being and to find beauty there.

Surrender is subtle. It's about being . . . not resisting. It's about being expansive and allowing something better, new possibilities. Surrender alleviates the anxiety of having to figure everything out and the fear of uncertainty. We can simply *be*. The feeling of surrender is like a sigh of relief, a weight lifted off your shoulders when you surrender control (which is ego). You'll float with the river, in the flow, and not swim against the current. Your spirit will guide you.

This is where synchronicity happens—the magic, the insights. Instead of freaking out, filling our time with busyness, or trying to *think* our way through it, we relax, breathe, and surrender to the bigger purpose of our health crisis, our life's journey, our soul's journey.

> You cannot discover new oceans unless you have
> the courage to lose sight of the shore.
> —André Gide

Letting Go

> When I let go of what I am, I become what I might be.
> —Lao Tzu

Once we accept and surrender, it quickly becomes clear how many things we do in life that, in the grand scheme of things, are distracting us from healing.

When your health crisis limits your physical/mental ability, it's time to let go of what no longer serves you (or that which you can no longer do). This makes room for that which matters, creating a void where new opportunities can grow.

What can I remove from my life to make room for something better, more healing? What can I let go of? What no longer serves me? Where do I feel as though I'm swimming upstream? If it doesn't bring me joy, is it necessary? Am I spending time with inspiration-sucking activities or people?

Ask the questions. Make the list. Bless it, loosen your grip, and let go—gracefully.

> As we "loosen our grip," we effortlessly bring more grace to us as we enter into the organic flow of life.
> —Sandra Ingerman, *The Book of Ceremony*

Letting go creates space into which flows what you truly need to heal, what brings you bliss, and what allows your most authentic self to flourish.

> In the end, only three things matter: how much you loved,
> how gently you lived, and
> how gracefully you let go of things not meant for you.
> —Buddha

Time is the greatest, most precious gift. In today's culture, everything demands our time: people, work, technology, community commitments, social obligations, advertisers, and lots of bright, shiny objects vying for our attention. Another insightful question we can pose to, well, everything, is *Does it matter? If so, how much does it matter? What will it cost my health and lifeforce? Is it worth it?*

> The cost of a thing is the amount of what I
> will call life which is required to be exchanged
> for it, immediately or in the long run.
> —Henry David Thoreau, *Walden*

What can I let go of that will give me more time to heal? Bring more peace? Joy? Awareness? Time to spend in nature? Help me find purpose? When will I give myself permission if not now?

Liberation is letting go of anything that isn't essential or doesn't resonate with your authentic self, with your heart. Let it fall away. Move on.

> Move and the way will open.
> —Zen Proverb

Dysfunctional relationships, toxic jobs, others' opinions, our obsessions, addictions, busyness, perfectionism, and anything that doesn't serve you can in fact do the opposite and hold you hostage. Let go of such things and embrace simplicity so you can be free to embody this new, healthier chapter of your life.

The Cursed "Shoulds"

The key to better health is finding new opportunities that won't damage your health into which you can channel your energy, passion, and/or creativity. Banish the cursed "shoulds," which only make us feel bad. Make "want-tos" your priority. Illness is your permission slip to walk away (responsibly) from everything that isn't serving your best health in this moment.

In the past, I was a prisoner of *should*, a prison of my own making. While I've cultivated my awareness and worked to banish the shoulds, it requires—for me, and I'm guessing a lot of us—constant attention.

For example, I was doing really well at banishing the shoulds until COVID-19 lockdowns happened. I felt I *should* be doing something: cleaning closets, reorganizing my studio, etc. But what most of us needed during the pandemic was robust self-care: rest and time to process grief and a roller coaster of emotions. It occurred to me, *Ah, they're back, the cursed shoulds.* With this awareness, I pivoted, let go of shoulds, and chose self-care instead.

Banishing the shoulds from your life is a big step toward relieving suffering. Of course there are essential shoulds: we should file our taxes on time, take care of young children and pets, pay our bills, and honor our relationships. However, for the unhelpful, possibly unnecessary shoulds, I've found an effective exercise.

Exercise: Banishing Shoulds

Make a list of the shoulds bouncing around your brain. Examine each one and determine if it's possible—and in your health's best interest—to shift any of the shoulds into a want-to. Here's an example: from "I should finish cleaning off the kitchen table" to "I'm eager to clean off the table so I can set up my watercolor easel here." If you can reframe a should and come at it with a sense of fun, curiosity, enthusiasm, or play, then it's a pretty good bet it's in alignment with your self-care. If you can't, let it go.

What's no longer serving me? How am I holding myself hostage with forces I believe I have no control over? Examine those things and you may realize you do indeed have control over them—which ultimately means you can set yourself free.

> In the space of letting go, she let it all be.
> A small smile came over her face.
> A light breeze blew through her.

> And the sun and the moon shone forevermore . . .
> —Safire Rose, "She Let Go"

Let it all go . . . let go of outcomes, expectations, things no longer meant for you—objects and activities as well as people. Let go of old emotional patterns—feel, process, learn from them, then let them go . . . and be at peace.

When you get rid of these weeds, you'll make room for new seedlings to blossom into new possibilities. Letting go of what no longer serves you is the ultimate form of self-love and self-acceptance.

> Maybe the journey isn't so much about becoming anything. Maybe it's about unbecoming everything that isn't you, so you can be who you were meant to be in the first place.
> —Paulo Coelho

When we let go of what's not in our highest good, we can peel away the layers of what *isn't* truly us. In other words, letting go brings you closer to your most authentic self, to your beautiful *you*. There is only one you in the entire universe. Why not be your most authentic you?

This process is similar to sculpting a work of art: removal shapes the piece, and in life, the peace. As we let go of that which no longer serves us, we make room for magic, miracles, and enchantment in our lives.

Dropping "Hows"

One of the most difficult things to let go of is the expectation of exactly how things work out. Dropping the need to influence the "hows" is one of the surest routes to more peace and happiness.

Here's an example: before the disastrous disc rupture, I was an avid hiker. Today, I can only walk for about ten or fifteen minutes without agonizing pain. My intention is to be able to walk more than that . . . one day, whenever it happens. I have no expectation of how much and no deadline as to when. I live in the moment, disregarding the hows. By letting go of the hows, I have freedom from pressure and space to heal. I replaced hiking time with robust self-care and began to heal at a more accelerated pace.

Yes, have goals and keep track of progress metrics. But in the face of enormous health challenges, be gentle with yourself. Drop the hows.

THE DANCE OF TRANSFORMATION

This trifecta of acceptance, surrender, and letting go is a dance of transformation.

Since I was a teen, I've battled depression, except, oddly, not in these five years. I've had no major episode of depression despite being in the perfect storm for a major and lasting episode. I attribute it to this trifecta.

Acceptance, surrender, and letting go are healing. Don't stress yourself out by fighting your health crisis, trying to control every detail and outcome, or holding on to things no longer meant for you. Life is already stressful enough.

I'm learning that everything happens as it should, everything happens for a reason, and everything happens at the right time. Trust that and make peace with it, recognizing we heal faster and find inner peace and harmony when we don't fight it.

Go with the flow. That's my aspiration—and daily challenge.

To be otherwise is to be resistant to *what is*—and that disrupts the dance of transformation. What we resist persists—or as psychologist Carl Jung contended, "What you resist not only persists, but will grow in size."[66] Get rid of resistance—mentally, but also energetically and spiritually.

Resistance blocks the blessings. Drop the resistance by accepting your circumstances. Surrender and let go.

Here's a little ritual for aiding the process:

- Make a list of things you wish to let go of—people, places, jobs, activities, thoughts, false beliefs, shoulds, hows.
- As you review each item, bless it.
- Now go burn it in your fireplace or tear it up.
- Breathe deeply into that sense of freedom.
- Set your intention for healing. *What could fill the space left by things released?*
- How might your life improve as a result? Embody this feeling.
- *Believe* in your new life, and give thanks for it in advance.

Feel better? If not, keep working the process. Like so many things in life, it's like an onion with many layers to be stripped away.

20

SURROUNDED BY SHARKS: HOLDING ONTO HOPE

> When it rains, look for rainbows.
> When it's dark, look for stars.
>
> —Oscar Wilde

In my mid-twenties, after my divorce, a friend and I decided two weeks in Mexico would heal our broken hearts. Back then, the Yucatan still had dreamy undeveloped beauty and pristine beaches.

My friend met a nice businessman who took us sailing in the shimmering azure waters, and we spent a blissful day on the sugar-white beaches of Isla Mujeres enjoying ceviche and cervezas in a little palapa at the shore's edge, listening to The Beatles.

On the way back to Cancun, we stopped to snorkel Palancar Reef in the middle of the ocean channel. With land nowhere in sight, my friend and I jumped into the endless sea and snorkeled above the reef teeming with life.

I was a fish in the water, agilely swimming about, parrotfish nibbling at my fingers as I eyed a school of barracuda below. When I came up for air, everything had changed—big swells, six to eight feet high. As I crested one, I pivoted 360 degrees . . . no boat. I waited for the next swell. No boat. Next swell. Nada.

I bobbed about for a bit, shivering (from nerves, mostly). In the inky darkness below, I saw perhaps thirty nurse sharks, all eyes on me. It's important to mention here that as a marine biology major, I'd dived and snorkeled with docile sharks before. But here, with no tether, my snorkeling bestie and boat nowhere in sight, and a scary shark gang below, dread prickled down my spine.

Now what? How will this be okay? I can't swim to land. Heck, which direction is land? I treaded water with one arm held high in the air. You know, just in case my friend could see me. I was so lost and far from home. I thought it was over. Yep, I was pretty sure it was over.

Then . . . I faintly heard a sputtering motor. Pretty soon I was plucked from the water, rescued from the dark, vast sea. All because I didn't give up hope. You can't keep your arm up high in the air and give up hope at the same time. Holding your hand high requires energy, like holding onto hope requires energy.

When my disc ruptured so disastrously years ago, I had a feeling of dread similar to the one that day in the waters off the Yucatan. At the time, a distant memory of that moment flickered into my mind. *I'm in deep water surrounded by menacing threats . . . I think it's over. What now? How will this be okay? Will I ever be okay?* Then a long-buried coping mechanism surfaced: *Keep holding your hand high and don't give up hope.*

Until the day you draw your last breath and die, you are alive.

Fully embody each day you're here.

Hold onto hope.

Every morning when I stretch, I raise my arms high in the air, a gesture of hope. This has become a metaphor for my healing journey. Never lose hope. When we have hope, we can plant seeds of health, water them with positive intentions, and reap the harvest of our dreams for a better life.

Becoming Fluent in Hope and Optimism

Sure, when life gives you lemons, make lemonade. A dollop of hope, like honey, sweetens the drink. When you're faced with a long, difficult convalescence, the key to survival is becoming fluent in hope and optimism. You may feel deep sadness, loss, pain, and overwhelm, but don't give up. Become fluent in hope. Commit yourself to it every day.

Studies have found hope is associated with "improved physical and mental health, relationships, functional status, and coping."[67]

So how do you become fluent in hope and optimism?

- Face fears.
- Love your life.
- Live fully in this present moment.
- Find your passion—what lights you up.
- Develop grit—your passion plus perseverance.
- Foster resilience—the capacity to spring back into shape.
- Follow your life's purpose, your unique gifts, your calling.

For me, every day I realize I'm not finished living the life of my dreams yet, even though the dreams continue to be redefined along this road to healing. Long before I became debilitated physically, I found the passions that made the time fly and my work that gives me purpose and makes the world a better place. I found my unique gifts and mastered them (art, photography, music, writing, my work). This gives me hope in every moment.

If you don't know what your passion and purpose are or if you didn't achieve mastery by the time you had a health crisis, focus on finding just one thing you love that gives your life meaning and makes the hours sail by as you're happily in the flow. Keep doing that. Or find something else. Obviously, the more positive the pursuit, the better.

> I dwell in possibility.
> —Emily Dickinson

The one thing that gives you hope is the thing you must latch on to. It will pull you out of the abyss of despair. What you encourage will wake up in you. Help it along. Accept the invitation. Fan the flames of hope every day, and you'll become fluent.

Resiliency and a sense of soul purpose carry us onward in spite of our health setbacks. *What did you come here to do? What's your passion? What's your purpose?*

Success—and a new life—can come at any age, despite ability limitations, if you hold onto hope and optimism.

Leafing through my journal of those early days following the disc rupture, I glimpse rays of hope. I emailed a friend, "It's a glorious spring day here, and a stellar blue jay makes a nest outside our bedroom window (from where I work and live these days). It's a reminder for me to build a new nest, nurture the eggs (or my health, as it were), then watch the little hopes grow stronger and eventually fly."

Choose hope in every moment. Commit that you'll remain optimistic and hold on to hope.

With a heart full of hope, you must believe your future will be better than where you are now. To succeed requires hope but also a plan (more on that in the chapters ahead).

> "Hope" is the thing with feathers -
> That perches in the soul -
> And sings the tune without the words -
> And never stops - at all -
> —Emily Dickinson

21

COURAGEOUSLY DARE TO HEAL

> Life shrinks or expands in proportion to one's courage.
>
> —Anaïs Nin

Courage is not the absence of fear. Having courage on the healing journey means we embrace our fragile humanness, face our fears head-on, and overpower them with love and hope. With courage, we can heal.

When you harness your courage, you'll find you're powerful beyond measure. Your body's healing ability is immense. Everything you need is inside you—to navigate the rough terrain of this challenging journey, your courageous heart is your compass.

Here's the trick: we must get some distance from daily suffering by taking an aerial view of our health condition as a pathway to more robust, transformational personal and spiritual development.

Bill Burnett and Dave Evans remind us, "A well-designed life is a marvelous portfolio of experiences, of adventures, of failures that taught you important lessons, of hardships that made you stronger and helped you know yourself better, and of achievements and satisfactions."[68] In other words, failures and hardships are key elements of the journey that shape a successful life. Stop cursing your health challenges and, with courage, lean into them as opportunities to make you stronger and know yourself better.

Every quest brings personal growth. Joseph Campbell wrote, "The grail quest often is set in a wasteland. It's in the bleakest, darkest, distressing times we discover our power, assume the mantle of the warrior or goddess in our own Hero's Journey, discover magnificent interior castles . . . and come out the other side stronger and whole. We realize we're not searching the external world for the holy grail, but that we are the treasure we've been seeking."[69]

Finding the treasure—you—takes enormous courage. This discovery requires a fundamental shift in perception: *you are not a victim of your health condition*. It's an intrinsic part of your life's journey that's calling you to be more courageous, vulnerable, and compassionate with yourself. It's part of your life purpose now. And with it comes deep healing. Dare to heal. Find the blessings in the challenges. Trust the journey.

In my situation, the spinal disc rupture itself lasted mere minutes. Yet, like most accidents and illnesses, the fear, pain, suffering, and loss could have lasted a lifetime. In those early days when courage was missing in action and my fears consumed me, I recommitted to being a fierce warrior-heroine who would not let this health crisis defeat my spirit. Instead I courageously dared to heal. The quest has permanently changed me . . . for the better. I emerged stronger and more empowered than I ever imagined I could be.

With every chapter ahead, you'll continue to grow your courage. In the meantime, here is an affirmation:

My healing journey is integral to my life's purpose.
I dare to heal. My body knows how.
I am listening. I am fierce. I am courageous.
You got this!

SUFFERING TO THRIVING

When courage comes alive, imprisoning walls become frontiers of new possibility, difficulty becomes invitation, and the heart comes into a new rhythm of trust and sureness.
—John O'Donohue

22

EVER ALWAYS GRATITUDE

> Gratitude unlocks the fullness of life. It turns what we have into enough, and more. It turns denial into acceptance, chaos to order, confusion to clarity. . . .
> It turns problems into gifts, failures into successes, the unexpected into perfect timing, and mistakes into important events. . . . Gratitude makes sense of our past, brings peace for today, and creates a vision for tomorrow.
>
> —Melodie Beattie

If you came to my house, you'd see a yellowing piece of paper on the refrigerator inscribed with the above quotation. It's been there for over a decade. A friend gave it to me during a particularly rough patch when I'd forgotten the wisdom of Melodie Beattie books I'd read decades prior. Her words not only got me through bad days but they have also benefitted my entire life.

As I look in the rearview mirror of this lifelong healing journey, I recognize every word of that quotation as truth. Go ahead, read it again. Put it on your own refrigerator or wherever you'll see it daily. Take the words to heart and watch your life transform.

Decades of daily gratitude practice have improved my mental and physical health and helped me create a safe, nurturing space to ride out any storm or lengthy holding pattern. When we live from a place of gratitude—despite our health challenges—we can find contentment, peace, and harmony.

How can we be happier? By being more grateful for what already is.

Turns out, gratitude is a powerful vibration—and a proven mood booster. One study shows that "training yourself to be more thankful can help people to feel better and increase mental resilience."[70] This makes sense because gratitude displaces negativity. Test it for yourself: you cannot be grateful and also angry, fearful, or self-pitying at the same time. Not possible. When your heart is brimming with gratitude, there's no room for negativity to creep in.

Gratitude transformed my life. It banished negative worries. Depression lifted. I found the silver lining of what I'd previously seen as problems. I became magnetic, attracting more good things into my life. Despite being disabled by pain and mobility issues, I've never been more grateful for my life, abundance, and good health.

Making a Habit of Giving Thanks

Here's a popular Zen saying—"How we do one thing is how we do everything." Building a gratitude practice means infusing all your activities throughout your life with awareness and appreciation. My practice evolved in four stages.

Whispers

For most of my life, my gratitude practice involved giving thanks upon waking in the morning and again at night before slumber. I call these thanks "whispers" because I speak them quietly to myself. I mostly expressed gratitude for the good stuff, especially the people who encouraged, held space, showed up, and remained present through the bad times.

Lists
At particularly difficult times, I stepped up my practice by regularly making lists of ten-plus things for which I was deeply thankful. Once, at an especially dismal point, I challenged myself to find more than one hundred reasons to be most grateful. It was a refreshing tonic to easily complete that list.

Daily Journal
Bigger shifts began to occur a couple of decades ago when I committed to keeping a daily gratitude journal. Some days I could find only one thing to be grateful for, but most days there were more. My gratitude journal keeps me accountable for sustaining this daily practice and keeps me focused on what matters. In moments of doubt or setbacks, looking back on my daily entries reminds me of how very blessed I am.

Perpetual Gratitude
The real game-changer happened about a year after my spinal collapse. Flat on my back for months on end, I began to understand how people could become old and bitter. One day I simply committed to living from a state of perpetual gratitude instead. This means taking nothing for granted and being unconditionally grateful for every occurrence on my healing journey, no matter how bad it might seem at first.

No matter what happens, be grateful for it and bless it. Yes, this means being grateful for the accident or disease before it transforms your life with new opportunities. Be grateful for loved ones who walk out of your life because now there's room for true friends who will stand by you through thick and thin. Be grateful for being housebound because of the time for contemplation and fresh insights that isolation and solitude allow. *How can I appreciate everything—"good" and "bad"? How is my healing journey a blessing?*

The above steps form a simple four-part tool. Is it easy? Well, certainly not at first. It's human nature to habitually react to things, labeling them as *good* or *bad*. At first, there may be too much anger, fear, or disappointment to find a scintilla of gratitude. Yet as we become aware of our minds reacting to things, we can begin to create a new way of responding. In time, muscle memory kicks in and your new gratitude habit becomes a way of life—a new operating system, if you will.

Mastering Gratitude

Like anything requiring muscle, mastering gratitude requires practice—as if we were aiming to become an Olympic athlete or a virtuoso musician. To achieve mastery of most skills requires ten thousand hours of practice.[71] While athletes and musicians also require innate talent, gratitude can be practiced by anyone.

Gratitude is a verb. What I mean is gratitude isn't the static list of things you're grateful for (i.e., nouns). Gratitude is action, a way of *be*-ing. *How can I live in a state of perpetual gratitude?* I count my blessings here and there while engaged in everyday activities: in line at the store, stuck in traffic, folding laundry, showering, making tea.

The more you live in this heart space of deeply felt, overflowing, unending gratitude, the more peace will permeate your life. Don't take my word for it—it's been scientifically proven: gratitude actually rewires your brain, making you happier and leading to better health and well-being.[72] That's why for thousands of years, across many cultures, gratitude has been a way of life.

Exercise: Gratitude

If you're new to the gratitude practice, this will get you started. Every morning upon waking before your feet hit the floor, again every evening when your head hits the pillow, and as often in between as possible, do the following:

- Name what you're most grateful for.
- Allow your heart to swell with gratitude.

- Feel the gratitude expand beyond your heart, into every pore.
- Let it permeate your room, your home, your community, your world.
- Hold onto this feeling as you go about your day.

This is a powerful practice. The more deeply—and often—you feel gratitude, the more powerful the peace and transformation. Embodying gratitude is good medicine. Here's my mantra:
In this moment, I am grateful for everything.
I have no complaints.

When You're Not Feeling It

We all have days when we're in a bad place. Perhaps we're utterly overwhelmed by a new diagnosis. Or exasperated by a perceived lack of progress in healing. Or full of anger. It's profoundly important to be patient and identify something, however small, for which to be thankful.

For instance, days after my debilitating disc rupture, my only activity was walking six steps to the bathroom and then back to bed (in searing pain and tears, cursing like a sailor). What could I possibly have had to be thankful for? A results-oriented overachiever at heart, I began to pay attention to the tiniest improvement. For months there was none. I couldn't see a future. Nonetheless, day in and day out, I gave thanks for being alive (and not any worse), for my husband's love and care, for friends who visited with groceries and meals, and for our lovely bedroom windows framing towering cedar trees. That's it. And that's a lot.

After a few months, I got up to fifty steps a day. Several months later, I could prop myself up in bed for ten minutes a day. After a year and a half, I could stand in the kitchen for ten minutes to make a salad or cup of tea. Then doctors permitted me to drive one mile into town to the pharmacy. I was ecstatically grateful for these freedoms.

My point is that even in the worst situations, finding gratitude for minuscule progress—or for simply being alive—brings peace and comfort.

> I have sometimes been wildly, despairingly, acutely miserable, racked with sorrow, but through it all I still know quite certainly that just to be alive is a grand thing.
> —Agatha Christie

Exercise: Advanced Gratitude

I look back on all the challenges of my healing journey with deep gratitude for their gifts of wisdom. Perhaps you too have reached this point in your journey?

If you don't already have a gratitude practice, beginning now will help you move from suffering to thriving.

Seeds of magic can be found in contemplating some advanced gratitude questions and meditations:

- How can I be grateful daily for the lessons on this healing journey?
- What is the silver lining of my healing crisis?
- (If you're struggling here, ask a trusted friend or family member to help identify what the silver lining might be. For me, it happened in one moment. I realized how deeply this could transform the trajectory of my life: I could allow my health crisis to depress me, or I could find the silver lining—and be wholly grateful for the journey.)

I leaned into gratitude, and it has transformed my soul. I realize it might sound unbelievable, but I'm eternally grateful for this healing journey, even the worst bits. I bless it and welcome its lessons of transformation. *Thank you, health issues, for opening the doors of opportunity that will transform my health and life.*

23

FEAR VS. LOVE

> Fear is the cheapest room in the house.
> I would like to see you living in better conditions.
>
> —Hafiz

It's human nature to be afraid. Ultimately, fear exists to keep us safe. It's a hardwired, ancient emotion—a survival mechanism from the age of *T. rex*. It served our prehistoric ancestors well, but in modern times? Not so much. Our everyday fears are (usually) not fanged and clawed, but a missed work deadline, computer crash, or scary health diagnosis can elicit the same fight, flight, or freeze response as a saber-toothed tiger in hot pursuit. Research tells us this kind of fear response can actually hasten physical and mental disease.

Worry is an extension of fear. When we face a health crisis, there are oh so many fears and worries over future uncertainty: *What will become of me? Will my ailment worsen? Will my pain become unbearable? Will I lose my mobility? Will I lose my mind? Will I lose my will to live? Will I die prematurely? Will my partner leave me? Will my friends forget me? Will I lose my job and face financial ruin? Will my kids be embarrassed by me?*

Fear seeps into your mind and rattles the cage of your body. Fear can immobilize you and lead to a downward spiral of stress, anxiety, anger, bitterness, a closed heart, and depression. When fear becomes a continuous background emotion, we need to choose a new way to be in the world.

Fear and love cannot coexist in the same moment. Thus an effective and beautiful way to conquer fear is with love. Buddhist nun Pema Chödrön teaches that everything we do in life comes from a perspective of either love or fear. When we look on ourselves, our relationships, our life situations, and our world with love—not fear—it changes everything.[73] Every day, in every moment, we have a choice: we can choose to take the path of love (e.g., happiness, gratitude, openness, sharing, celebration) or embody fear (anger, intolerance, struggle, shutting down).

Choose Love over Fear

> If you take all your fears, one by one, make a list of them, face them, decide to challenge them, most of them will vanish.
> —Anaïs Nin

People often ask how I maintain a positive attitude despite my health challenges. I don't allow fear to be in the driver's seat. That is not to say I'm fearless. But I do *face* fear almost every day—because it shows up every day. When we face fear, it no longer has power over us. Otherwise, what we resist (fear) persists (more fear). Let's drop the resistance by replacing fear with love.

We can diminish fear by showing up. Find a comfortable, safe place, open your journal, and practice the following steps:

- **Expose your fear.** Ask, *What are my fears?*
- **Drill down.** *What's at the root of this?* You might be afraid of people making fun of you, but perhaps you're really afraid of being alone. A fear of everything chang-

ing in your life might be rooted in a fear of losing control. If you listed several fears, are they rooted in the same basic fear, such as loss?

- **Face it.** Facing fear takes away its power. Next time fear grabs you, take a deep breath, recognize it for what it is, and choose not to allow it to put down roots. With a sense of inquisitiveness, face it, engage it, and get to know it better. *Fear, why are you in the driver's seat? How do you serve me?*

- **Assess it.** *Is my fear rational? Have I blown it out of proportion? What's the worst that could happen? Where is it holding me back? Is it deflated now simply because I faced it?*

- **Reframe it.** *This is only a fear. The truth is _____.*

- **Choose love instead.** Fill fear's void with love. *How can I harness my fear as something positive? How can I replace fear with a more loving thought, decision, or action? What can I love about my life or health? What can I be grateful for or celebrate?*

> I've been absolutely terrified every moment of my life, and I've never let it keep me from doing a single thing I've wanted to do.
> —Georgia O'Keeffe

When I was diagnosed with spinal diseases in my twenties, doctors told me I'd be in a wheelchair by my thirties. As you might imagine, I was frightened and depressed. Then it dawned on me: I was suffering every day as if it had already happened. I was letting fear steal my peace.

I decided I wouldn't "own" that prognosis by living from a place of fear. I didn't let it consume me. I decided I would find another way. I faced the fear and took the wind out of its sails. Decades later, I'm not wheelchair-bound. Let that sink in. I suppose it could happen someday, but I resolve not to give this fear any energy or power over me. I live as fully as possible with utter disregard for this fear.

One of the best ways to get a handle on your fears is to practice gratitude throughout your day, every day. If you're living from a place of gratitude (a form of love), there's no room for fear. If your heart is full of gratitude, fear can't take hold and carry you away to its dark place.

Although I was once fearful of future possibilities, today my spirit is a mountain—courageous, indomitable. When we cultivate a habit of facing and examining our fears, we diminish them and build more courage. It is profoundly empowering to stare down fear. Shine a light on it, and it evaporates. When you face your fears, you'll have found your courage. As we learned a few chapters back, on the healing journey, it's essential to fully inhabit your courage.

When we face fears, we step out to the precipice where our dreams can take flight. We embody fierce bravery, courage, and confidence. Decide right now that you won't let your fears defeat you. Embrace the unknown.

> In our culture, there is so much fear of the unknown that we would rather compromise our physical and emotional health.
> —Marcela Lobos

24

WONDER-FILLED

> Miracles happen every day; change your perception of what a miracle is and you'll see them all around you.
>
> —Jon Bon Jovi

Every day is an opportunity to observe miracles, magic, and mystery, especially when we're mindful about recognizing—and celebrating—them.

I'm filled with wonder and awe by everyday miracles:

- Earth is speeding around our sun star at sixty-seven thousand miles per hour while spinning on its axis at one thousand miles per hour.

- Our solar system is hurtling through the universe at about four hundred and forty-eight thousand miles per hour. Even at this rapid speed, the solar system would take about two hundred and thirty million years to travel all the way around the Milky Way.[74]

- The delicate balance of sun, rain, and oxygen not only makes life possible but also enables Earth to be our perfect, complete life support system.

- 8.7 million species of plants and animals inhabit Earth, each one with a unique, essential role.

- Our human bodies function in an amazing way.

- Of course, I'm awestruck by newborn babies, puppies, kittens, and butterflies.

In these modern times, we're all doing way too much. Then a physical or mental ailment is layered on top of all that. From this (often depressing) point of view, our eyes may dim to the magic, miracles, and mystery of each day. It's easy to get lost in a rut of not remembering they're always here waiting for us—if only we pause, disconnect from our technology, step out into the world, and open our eyes to the awe and enchantment of life. It's visible everywhere: birds in flight, the splendor of the seasons, trees communicating through subterranean fungi networks, the creation of new life everywhere we turn, on and on. Take this to heart:

I celebrate this day in awe of the miracles, magic, and mystery of life. I am open to wonder and awe.

As it turns out, awe is good for your health: "Experiencing awe over time could potentially have long-term health benefits."[75]

There are many books on the wonders of nature, everyday enchantment, mystery, and such, so I won't cover that territory here. But let's spend a moment exploring how we can rekindle our sense of wonder and awe:

- If you're physically able, get out into nature. Walk on a beach, hike in the woods, sit in the park, or go to your backyard. Observe everything from the grand vistas to the wee world mostly hidden from the untrained eye.

- Stargaze—watch for falling stars and identify the planets.

- Follow the daily journey of the moon's phases; observe the tides.

- Learn something new and fascinating to you—perhaps the secret life of trees, the myriad undersea creatures inhabiting our vast oceans, the plight of the bees and polar bears, quantum physics . . . you get the idea.
- Live your life in tune with the seasons.
- Watch a program about faraway lands and their wildlife or about our galaxy.
- Plant a garden (or a windowsill garden) and watch it grow.

The point is to find something that speaks to you and get curious. Look at it with wonder as you did when you were little. Make it a daily practice. Let your intuition be your guide.

Never lose your sense of curiosity. Never stop asking questions. Never stop learning. Being wonder-filled is good for your health.

> The beginning of our happiness lies in the understanding that life without wonder is not worth living. What we lack is not a will to believe but a will to wonder.
> —Abraham Joshua Heschel

25

RX: LAUGHTER

> Laughter, and a lot of it, is the right response
> to the things which drive us to tears.
>
> —Seneca

You've heard before—and Mayo Clinic research now confirms it—laughter is the best medicine. As important as a good cry, laughter has an essential role in healing and coping. Myriad books explore how people have cured chronic illnesses (even cancer) through laughter.

Turns out having a laugh relaxes our muscles, releases endorphins, alleviates stress, strengthens our social relationships, and brings big doses of oxygen into the bloodstream—all of which promote your body's healing response. Dr. Amit Sood writes, "Research shows laughter provides a good physical workout, generates mental relaxation, lowers blood pressure and pain, and even improves immunity. You're 30 times more likely to laugh in good company than alone. Further, the more you laugh with others rather than at someone, the greater the health benefit."[76]

Additionally, laughter has "physical, psychological, spiritual, and relational benefits. It is the cost-free medicine that can release endorphins helping us feel good, exercise our muscles and breathing like yoga, help us lighten moods and cope with problems more readily, and strengthen social bonds."[77] There's even something called laughter meditation.

Experiencing humorous entertainment lifts the spirits and our health. (Conversely, watching entertainment that brings you down or is violent will bring down your health response.)

Smiling has positive health benefits too. "It lifts our mood, as well as the moods of those around us . . . It can even lengthen our lives."[78] Smiling boosts the immune system—it's called psychoneuroimmunology.

A light heart and peaceful spirit are essential for good health. Cultivating a sense of humor, ease of laughter, bright smile, and playful spirit is good medicine we can weave into every day.

> To succeed in life, you need three things: a wishbone, a backbone, and a funny bone.
> —Reba McEntire

26

SPARKLING RESILIENCE

> Grief and resilience live together.
>
> —Michelle Obama, *Becoming*

Resilience is our capacity to bounce back quickly from adversity and setbacks like physical, mental, or emotional health challenges. We build it up by facing obstacles and loss with courage—all the while growing confident that we are stronger than we realize. It's worth building your resilience muscle because resilience gives us endurance to get through the healing journey—especially when facing long-term chronic conditions.

How do we endure health setbacks yet remain resilient? My practice is this: live mindfully one moment to the next from the highest consciousness, hope, and optimism possible. Live in much the same way as you'd climb a mountain—mindful of every step, all senses alive in every moment. We must remain optimistic we'll reach the summit.

The challenge, of course, is how to bring robust mindfulness and heady optimism into every moment of our daily lives despite trying circumstances. We learned a few chapters ago that when we accept our situation, acknowledge loss, surrender to what is, let go of what no longer serves us, and appreciate the journey, we build resilience. Resilience is a learnable skill.

Just as we pack the essentials in our mountain climbing adventure knapsack, The Thriving Toolkit—the final part of this book—packs essential tools for building your resilience.

Scaling the Mountain of Life

> Rock bottom became the solid foundation
> on which I rebuilt my life.
> —J.K. Rowling, *Very Good Lives*

I've always had the mindset that the bigger the goal, the bigger the blessing. Yet at the beginning of the healing journey, we must have the patience to start with baby steps. After all, when you were an infant, you had to crawl and then take baby steps before you could become adept at running or dancing, right?

> If you knew of a spectacular mountain that was very, very tall, yet climbable. And if it was well-established that from its peak, you could literally see all the love that bathes the world, dance with the angels, and party with the gods. Would you curse or celebrate each step you took as you ascended it?
>
> Righto!
> Life is that mountain and each day a step.
>
> Perspectives change everything,
> The Universe
>
> —Mike Dooley, *Manifesting Change*

As you know all too well, there are peaks and valleys on the healing journey. When you get to the pinnacle, it's a great high. From there you can see the brilliant light—your future—on the horizon.

Getting to the pinnacle usually means spending time in the shadowlands and at rock bottom. Everything in life is incremental. If you aim to reach the summit, your big goal, you must set incremental goals along the way. Focused micro-goals and micro-disciplines will help you work tenaciously and productively toward progress.

Every step of the journey—through successes and failures—helps build resilience.

> It is impossible to live without failing at something, unless you live so cautiously that you might as well not have lived at all
> —in which case, you fail by default.
> —J.K. Rowling, *Very Good Lives*

In my career, I describe myself as a goal-driven, results-oriented professional. Yet when faced with the enormity of healing from the disastrous disc rupture, for the first couple of months I didn't set any goals for myself. Then there were baby-step goals (e.g., sit up in bed by 2 p.m.; walk eleven steps from bed to the bedroom door). It wasn't only the searing pain (I howled after the first few steps)—I literally couldn't walk.

Epic failure, I thought. Yet I kept trying. Baby step by baby step, I learned to sit, stand, and walk again.

A friend told me, "Baby steps are okay because at least you're vertical and there's hope!" At that low point, I needed this message.

> Success is the ability to go from failure to failure without losing enthusiasm.
> —Unknown

Keep bouncing back. Hold onto your enthusiasm.

Fail your way forward. Failures can lead you to set new, ultimately more achievable goals. New goals are vital for our physical improvement as well as mental health.

Ready, Set, Goals

It's important to chart your progress so you can see where you've been and how much you've improved. Create something like this for yourself:

Time since rupture	*Two Weeks* Activity/Day	*Six Months* Activity/Day
Walking	only to the bathroom	two hundred steps/day
Standing	0	5 minutes
Sitting in a chair	0	0
Showering	0	Yes!

Because of the unique nature of your health condition, you'll have different goals. *What basic activities are affected by your illness/injury? What are the current thresholds on each activity (in minutes, hours, number of reps, etc.)? How can you structure a healing environment around these? What reminder(s) do you need (posted on the refrigerator, bathroom mirror, journal)? What are your big goals? What micro-goals will help you get there?* Chart your incremental progress at regular intervals.

Today, start where you are and give yourself permission to take baby steps. Eventually you'll persevere and push past whatever stands in your way. With dogged determination, consistent effort. and grit, you'll build your resilience muscle. Be content with incremental progress toward your big goals without time-limited pressures. You'll get there.

Honor your accomplishment by celebrating victories—large or small, life-changing or not. Do the happy dance or simply bask in the glow of achievement. Reward yourself with something as traditional as cake and champagne or some pampering self-care: a massage or acupuncture treatment, or perhaps a treat you've had your eyes on (new pj's anyone?) or that invests in your achievement (walking shoes? yoga mat?).

To envision your way forward, keep goals in play that are aimed at improving your circumstances and keeping hope alive. The goal-setting process looks something like this:

1. Set the big goal.
2. Break the big goal down into incremental chunks: micro-goals.
3. Achieve the incremental goal and ask, *Then what happens? And then what?*
4. Set a more ambitious incremental goal.
5. Fail—and learn why it failed.
6. Revise a more achievable incremental goal or work-around.
7. Master your incremental goal and achieve your big goal.
8. Celebrate (don't skip this).
9. Repeat.

What's your goal? Write it down and track it like this:

Goal	Date Set	Target Date	Success/ Failure	Date Achieved	What I Learned	Do I Need a Work-Around?	What's Next?

This process taught me a lot about myself and my spine. Almost every basic activity—walking, standing, sitting—is considered a high-impact no-no for me. Yet I went from only walking fifty to two hundred steps per day at the end of the first year to walking three thousand–plus steps in year five. I've gone from not being able to stand up at all to standing fifteen minutes or so. I could barely walk to the kitchen; now, every few months, I can go for a ten-to-fifteen–minute walk outdoors.

Although these are far from normal activities and nothing compared to the hiking and countless activities I did pre-rupture, I celebrate these achievements—and continue to set ever-bigger goals.

I've also learned a valuable skill: managing expectations. I've accepted I'll never ride a horse again. Or downhill ski. Or ride my bike. And I'm okay with it all. I look back on these activities with fond memories but place no expectation on experiencing them in the future.

Successfully managing expectations means being okay with *any* outcome. When discussing inner peace with a group of his students, spiritual teacher J. Krishnamurti said, "This is my secret . . . I don't mind what happens."[79]

I hope my situation will change. But it might not. At moments like this, it's vital to hit the reset button. Reframe. Recalibrate.

Hey, if there's a medical miracle and one day I can ride my bike again—or a horse—or walk ten thousand steps without destroying my back, it's all icing on the cake. But for now, I don't mind what happens. I'll focus on robust self-care and my new dreams.

Facing Setbacks with Grace

We have every expectation to get well. Friends and family cheerily say "Get better!" and "Hope you make a speedy recovery!" But what happens when months and years go by and we aren't better?

With chronic health crises, there will be setbacks. The unwanted dance of illness is one step forward and two steps back—if we're lucky, because we recognize it could just as easily be one step forward and six steps back. Or worse.

In this part of the journey, I've introduced you to the qualities of a thriving spirit:

- acceptance, surrender, and letting go

- hope
- courage
- gratitude
- love
- awe
- laughter
- resilience

We've looked at some helpful practices to get you started, but now it's time to start restructuring your life around the practices that will keep you in that thriving spirit space.

> Once you make a decision,
> the universe conspires to make it happen.
> —Ralph Waldo Emerson

PART 6

THE THRIVING TOOLKIT

To restore your health, find joy, and be at peace, you'll need every tool in the Toolkit.

Whether you're an artist, woodworker, construction expert, surgeon, or family cook, you know how important it is to have the best tools for the job. What follows is your Toolkit of holistic strategies for navigating the journey from suffering to thriving. While each tool can produce benefits, the whole truly is greater than the sum of its parts.

Integrate these transformative tools into your life, and you'll see an internal shift toward more resilience, well-being, peace, harmony, and joy.

Reading about it doesn't count as experience. To heal, we must practice with our tools. Try it all. What works for you? Healing is personal, and there's no magic bullet. Every individual responds differently. That's why it's important to try different modalities. I encourage you to play super sleuth and see how these practices might fit into your healing journey—as needed or as part of a regular practice. Hold an intention to heal, and keep an open mind.

These pages hold liberation from your suffering.

27

TRANSFORMATION: SITTING IN DARKNESS LIKE A CATERPILLAR

> When you come out of the storm you won't be the same person who walked in. That's what this storm's all about.
>
> —Haruki Murakami, *Kafka on the Shore*

I enjoy celebrating the winter solstice as a gateway of transformation, a time to hunker down for the winter, weather its storms, hibernate in the darkness in anticipation of light, and pause to incubate new ideas. In winter we learn that change is the foundation for growth. The frozen landscape appears barren, yet beneath the surface, the unseen earth is transforming, patiently awaiting spring to explode into life.

If we can recognize and accept our healing journey as a winter of the soul—urging us to sit patiently in its darkness, discomfort, and uncertainty, hibernating inward—we will discover the seeds of new life incubating beneath the surface. Then one day, from brokenness and vulnerability we emerge transformed, with grace, blossoming into new life.

A wonderful Inuit word captures the essence of this moment: *qarrtsiluni*—sitting together in darkness, perhaps expectantly (e.g., waiting for something to happen or to "burst forth"); the strange quiet before a momentous event.[80] New life comes from this fecund darkness: human life in the womb's darkness, seeds deep within the earth, and yes, the qarrtsiluni of your healing journey.

Darkness and uncertainty are where the caterpillar hangs out: it feels like the end of its world until it emerges from darkness a breathtaking butterfly—a light, joyful thing of beauty. It might be difficult to see now, but you too will transform into an ever more beautiful shining soul.

Embracing the Magic in Uncertainty

> Everything changes and nothing stands still.
> —Heraclitus

It's human nature to want to banish uncertainty—we plan goals, reach milestones, and cross life experiences off the list. But when we can relax and embrace uncertainty in dark times of transition, such as the healing journey, we'll learn it's where the magic is.

Inside the chrysalis, the caterpillar's body completely dissolves into a soup of nutrients, the magic sauce that creates this magnificent new butterfly creature! Before transformation occurs, there's the holding pattern. We ask "What's next?" but cannot foresee the metamorphosis in store for us. The sooner you learn to embrace uncertainty with a sense of curiosity, wonder, and patience, the more peace you'll find. The cocoon can be ugly and dark inside. Yet what emerges—at the right time, not a minute sooner—is beautiful.

Trust this alchemy of transformation. Trust that something beautiful will emerge from this darkness of your healing journey. Trust your new story, gestating in the dark.

Mythic Shape-Shifters

> Change is inevitable, but transformation
> is by conscious choice.
> —HeatherAsh Amara, *The Toltec Path of Transformation*

As you might guess, my own story is a butterfly-fairy-tale-shape-shifting transformation kind of story. As with any emerging butterfly, it has not been an easy metamorphosis. In one decade, I lost my job, started my business, and grieved the early deaths of treasured friends. Then the catastrophic spinal disc rupture left me disabled for nearly five years. During that time, we were evacuated twice due to wildfires, then the roads washed out and left our community stranded for many months. So my husband had to live in another town on weekdays for work at a time when I relied upon him most.

But everything worked out—in fact, something better has emerged. Who I was then is not who I am today, and I couldn't be more thrilled about it! Like the caterpillar in the chrysalis, I've emerged with wings. By shape-shifting, I learned to transcend and fly untethered out of darkness, soaring above it with joy, freedom, courage, big dreams, and fierce, empowered confidence.

All healing—the transition from sickness to health—is transformation. I believe our health crises emerge in our lives to quiet the loud thrum of the world so we can hear the heart's voice and soul's purpose. Sometimes we must leave behind the life we're living in order to be metamorphosed into a new world.

Whether you realize it or not, you too have embarked upon a mythic journey of transformation. Myths, folk tales, and fairy tales from many cultures are replete with shape-shifters in search of hidden treasures: self-exploration, deepening intuition and spirituality, creativity, reconnection with nature, or birthing a new life. We might discover this process is not in step at all with society, family, and/or work.

Then there's the ultimate form of shape-shifting: the epic journey of discovering and embodying your life purpose. Carl

Jung believed that right underneath your wound (be it physical, mental, or emotional) lies your individual gift or calling—what you were meant to manifest in this lifetime. We grow from our wounds. In other words, your healing journey can be the catalyst to growing into your life's purpose.

Exercise: The Butterfly Emerges

Here's an excerpt from one of my journal entries:

> **December 18, 2018—***The spark has returned to my eyes, passion to my soul, sense of purpose to my heart. I'm shape-shifting from my old life into these brand new beginnings!*

You too will emerge from the darkness—just as the caterpillar morphs into a butterfly, as the light of day follows the darkest night, as spring bursts forth from the dead of winter.

Once your transformation begins, you cannot go back to your previous life any more than the butterfly can crawl back into the chrysalis. What's more, you won't want to. A switch flips and you feel driven forward by passion, perhaps for something bigger than yourself.

Your healing journey offers a new lens through which to view your life's purpose—and it's the catalyst for achieving it.

What's your intention for your transformation? Have you contemplated your life's mission? Grab a pen and paper and make a list of what you were. Like the caterpillar, describe the end of your world as you knew it. Then make another list beside it of whom you wish to become. *Like a caterpillar with big dreams, what would you enjoy morphing into? What do you intend for the short term? What do you aspire to in your lifetime? What's your reason for being? How do you wish to contribute to humanity? What's your legacy? How do you wish to be remembered when you're gone?* Write the first thoughts that come to mind, and don't edit yourself. Follow your intuition and let it flow. This is healing.

SUFFERING TO THRIVING

My hope is that you'll listen deeply to these incantations and one day awaken to your new life, seeing yourself as if for the first time like the phoenix emerging from the fire.

28

WRITE A DIFFERENT ENDING

> Tell me, what is it you plan to do
> with your one wild and precious life?
>
> —Mary Oliver, "The Summer Day"

When I was young, my parents, younger sister, grandmother, and I would spend a couple of weeks each summer on road trips, venturing from our home in Western Pennsylvania to upstate New York, New England, and Canada. Our big green Rambler station wagon had a rumble seat in the far back—facing backward—and my parents thought it the perfect place for us arguing sisters. I never liked that rumble seat. Then, as now, I didn't enjoy looking back at where I'd been—only ahead toward places yet to be discovered.

As I grew older, my "never look back" attitude became a strongly rooted personality trait. When my health got rocky, it served me well: *don't look behind—you're not going that direction.*

The First Peoples of Australia tell us "the big stories are hunting the right people to tell them."[81] Every life has many stories. Sometimes our new story finds us through a health crisis. It helps to view a health condition—or whatever life throws at us—as a portal to a new story for our lives. We must "rewrite" our stories from a bird's-eye view and a place of curiosity about the future. The challenge is shifting from "Ugh, I have this dreaded ailment, and I can't believe I had to go through hell" to "I'm grateful to this health crisis for helping me to chart a new course on my life journey, find new dreams, reach my full potential, find my life purpose, achieve self-realization, and/or bask in inner peace."

For example, I've re-storied my life from "My health setbacks destroyed my wonderful life" to "My healing journey is part of the story I came here to tell." I've accepted this, surrendered to my calling, and no longer struggle against it. I've mined wisdom that will help me, and others, to thrive. It's a good story.

Ask the Right Questions

You've probably experienced the mind chatter I call the "what-ifs." *What if this happens to me? What if that happens? What if it's terrible?* It's easy to fall into a downward spiral. Let's turn it around by asking the right questions and, with your answers, writing a better ending for your story.

- What if I decide, right now in this moment, to fall in love with my future?
- What if I reinvent myself?
- What if I'm on the cusp of something *great*?
- What if there's a better way of doing this? (The answer is always *yes!*)

Exercise: You Are Here

Grab your journal and prepare to do more creating. Begin with the question "Where did it all begin?" Write a bit about the onset of your health crisis, how your life changed, and where you are today. Don't worry about grammar. No need to share this. Writing down the bones of it will help you gain clarity.

Get creative and write your story like a novel or fairy tale. *Is your ailment the villain? A dragon to slay or charm? What's the epic battle of your health catastrophe? Deep pain? Fear? Were your dreams crushed?*

By this point in your journey, maybe your loved ones are weary of listening to you. *What do you need to acknowledge in your own heart?* Share what you write with kindred spirits—or burn it as a cathartic offering. Either way, it's a doorway to healing.

If writing isn't your thing, draw or paint a map of your healing journey so far—beginning at "You are here." Then add to your entry as you read on.

Let Go of Your Old Story

Birds cannot fly if they hold tight to the branch. If your health crisis has radically changed your life, you might need to let go of your old life—temporarily or forever.

In looking for a new story to live by, I discarded the old story I'd embodied before the disabling disc rupture that included spending my summers happily traveling the world and my dream of one day living in France or Italy. I let it go, making room for *new* adventures.

Think of all the labels you've worn and the activities you did up until your health crisis—or struggle to hold onto now. *Can you let go of those that no longer fit in order to make room for something new and fulfilling?*

A Different Kind of What-If?

Instead of "Why did this happen to me?" and "When will this be over?" let's ask better questions:

- What can I learn from this experience? What's it trying to teach me?
- What's the opportunity for growth in this situation?

- How can I create a life of meaning?

As mentioned in Chapter 14, "Taking Inventory," another right question to ask is "What *can* I do?" (If you haven't already, now's a good time to do that exercise as it works synergistically with the questions above.)

Dare to dream a new life with a different ending where your ailment isn't holding you back. You'll find infinite possibilities when you ask, from a space of curiosity and hope, "Now what? What next? What if?"

For instance, "What if something wonderful is about to happen?" Ask and expect the good stuff! Remember, this isn't about sugarcoating or denial but intending your best possible life.

Over a decade ago, enthralled by this idea, I created an art collage with words that became my forever mantra:

Something wonderful is about to happen.

Wouldn't you know it, almost every day, something wonderful *does* happen!

Let's Dream

Think of your ailment as a course correction to your life journey so far. It's beckoning you to be nimble, dream a little, and find a new path. Imagine traveling a few years into your future. *What possibilities await you there? Can you see your happily ever after?* Don't worry about the details, just feel the happily ever after. *What makes it so?* Write, draw, or paint it. Then ask, "What step could I take to bring myself closer to it?"

What Kind of Wonderful?

As you break out of the label of your health crisis, give a title to your new life story, your aspirational dream. If you're physically disabled, perhaps your new story is *A Spiritual Adventure*, or *Destination: PhD*, or *My Mystic Life*. If you're experiencing cognitive decline, your new story might be *Living Every Moment Well*, *Savoring the Present*, or *Physical Shape-Up*. You get the idea. Visualize the destination. No change is possible without imagining it first.

WAYFINDING

Imagining your happy ending is the first step of your new beginning. Once you have a general idea of the new life you seek, let's explore how we get there from here. Wayfinding is simply mapping a new path forward step by step. As with planning any journey, it helps to ask the right questions.

- What boundaries can I push?
- What good things *could* happen?
- What new skills would I like to develop for my "new life"?
- What attributes—physical, mental, emotional, spiritual—would I like to cultivate?
- What personal development goals would I like to achieve?
- What can I let go of to make room for my new dreams?
- What steps can I take today? Next week? Next month?

Contemplate these questions, grab your journal, and write a different ending. Draw or paint your happy ending on your map. Get creative with it. It doesn't need to be perfect. Have fun imagining the infinite possibilities unfolding on the road before you. Nothing is set in stone. You can reimagine it all again tomorrow.

Cross the Chasm

Once you have an image of your desired destination, it's important to get from where you are now (point A) to where you're ultimately going (point B). Visualization is powerful for manifesting a bridge from your point A to point B.

- Find a comfortable, safe space where you won't be disturbed for at least ten minutes.
- Think about where you are today in your life (point A).
- Imagine the best possible outcome (point B) from the exercise above.
- How will you feel when you arrive at point B? Vividly feel the emotions. Feeling the "happily ever after" you seek is key to manifesting your new story.
- Now imagine a bridge you could easily cross to get to your new life. A little footbridge across a forest stream? A strong bridge across a river? A bridge adorned with flowers along a boardwalk through a meadow?
- Visualize crossing the bridge to your new life. How does it feel to get to the other side? Imagine the sights (balloons! confetti!), sounds (cheers!), and joy welling up within you.
- Believe with every fiber of your being that your new life is on the way to you.

Now take the first step, and simply do the best you can. You're on your way!

29

MONK MORNING

How we spend our days is, of course, how we spend our lives.

—Annie Dillard

Mornings often begin with a too-early alarm clock, fielding emails and text messages, checking the calendar to assess the breakneck schedule ahead, gulping coffee while glued to the news, going for a run, grabbing some breakfast, getting to work, or shuttling kids off to school.

It's not a peaceful start to the day, is it? Actually, it's the antithesis of the rest and recovery our bodies need when we're unwell.

Enter Monk Morning. Yes, it's a thing. Social media influencers extoll the virtues of their Monk Morning routines, but there's no one-size-fits-all formula. What matters is a morning routine to ease *you* into *your* day. We'll create one for your unique needs, abilities, life and health circumstances, and passions.

Do the most important things in life first.
The best thing you can do—
for yourself and those you love—
is to put your self-care at the top of the list
along with your personal development.

First let's look at my restorative, energizing Monk Morning that fits it into fifteen minutes or an hour, depending on available time.

- In the hypnopompic state between dreaming time and awakening, I recall my dreams, jot down details, and seek meaning there. Sometimes a poem whispers in my ear, and I catch it before it whizzes by in search of another poet.

- Still in bed, I slowly stretch and do a couple of physical therapy exercises to ease my spine into the day.

- Next it's gratitude practice and setting my intention for the day.

- I make a cup of golden milk and return to bed to rest (to push through the pain now would ruin the day), mindfully admiring the towering cedars and blue sky. Five or ten minutes is quite restorative.

- Now's a nice time to light some blue lotus incense, sage, palo santo, or a candle. As I do, I say a blessing of peace, love, and light for all sentient beings. I may read a page of something inspiring or close my eyes and do a visualization, or meditate on a mantra. The simple word *peace* is my go-to mantra on high-stress workdays.

- With a crystal in hand, I do a little Reiki, sometimes accompanied by Tibetan crystal bowls or meditation music. I do a quick body scan (see Chapter 36, "The Guided Journey"), noting areas of blocked energy. Then I run my energy, ground to the earth, and draw energy from Divine Source.[82]

- To signal the end of Monk Morning and the mindful beginning of my workday, I gently ring a Tibetan singing bowl tuned to the Sacral Chakra for energy and creativity.

After this intentional, soul-aligned ritual Monk Morning, I'm ready to approach my workday with clarity, focus, mindfulness, and calm.

Exercise: Design Your Own Monk Morning

Hopefully you can carve out at least ten minutes a day for Monk Morning—or Monk Evening, if it suits you better. The greater your time investment in your sacred practice, the bigger the dividends.

With the help of these targeted questions, ascertain what resonates with you:

- Before you jump out of bed, is there anything you'd like to do? Dream recall? Gratitude? Prayers? Stretching? Reiki? Yoga nidra?

- Ritual focuses the mind. What type of ritual might help signal the opening of a sacred space? A bell? A drumbeat? Tea? Essential oils? Incense? Candles? Sage? Palo santo? A religious ritual?

- What kind of music? Benedictine monks? Native American flute? Instrumental music? Chanting? New age music? Classical? Aim to create a positive vibe that sets the tone for your day.

- Does stillness make you feel good and give you energy? Seek out quiet meditation, prayer, or visualization (see Chapter 36, "The Guided Journey"). Read a page or two from a book that sets an inspiring, contemplative, or prayerful tone. Or set your intention for the day.

- If you prefer movement, consider a hike in nature, walking meditation, Qigong, Tai Chi, gardening, yoga (or chair yoga if you're physically compromised), or freeform dance. In fact, research recognizes dance's health-promoting benefits for the mind, body, emotions, and spirit.

- Would you prefer to block out time to channel creative ideas such as journaling, art, music, or poetry?

Start by selecting two or three activities you wish to explore. Tinker with your practice until it's in strong alignment with your mind, body, and spirit. After a week or more, contemplate *How has Monk Morning changed my life? Physical and/or mental health? Resilience? Outlook on the future? Stress level? Peace index?*

Be attentive and modify your Monk Morning to accommodate your changing energy levels. If your ritual feels stagnant, it's no longer in alignment with your current needs. Listen to your intuition. Play with it until you find the right flow of energy.

This is meant to be one of the handiest tools in your Toolkit for kick-starting your best possible, most healing day. Have fun with it!

Do it daily. One day it will become your practice, and you won't recall how you got by without it.

30

HEALING POWER OF ART

> Art is to console those broken by life.
>
> —Vincent van Gogh

Whether you're an artist or musician or believe you have no artistic talent at all, creative expression is essential for healing physically and mentally. Art is medicine. Even Western science agrees; a review of the literature on art and healing suggests that "Engagement with creative activities has the potential to contribute toward reducing stress and depression and can serve as a vehicle for alleviating the burden of chronic disease."[83] According to Ronit Fallek, a healing arts practitioner, studies show that engaging in any creative process is healing. Whether you make a simple drawing or collage, look at art or talk about it, creativity and the arts can help you

- express thoughts and emotions that can be hard to put into words
- lower stress and anxiety
- relax and feel calmer and happier

- connect with yourself on a deep level, no matter what you're going through
- find meaning in life experiences
- cope with grief and loss
- form new connections with others
- shift your focus away from pain or stressful thoughts to activities that are soothing, enjoyable, and fun
- create something unique that gives you a sense of pleasure and accomplishment[84]

What's more, music has been scientifically proven to keep your brain young and healthy.[85]

I find music and art to be beautiful healing ways to live from our heart centers and to discover that magic place of being in the flow. Doing something creative every day has been an essential element of my healing journey. Following the tug of ideas and bursts of inspiration—or simply noodling around—opens up pathways of discovery and deep healing.

You might be thinking, "I can't be creative right now; my health won't allow it," or "That's fine for you, but I'm not a creative person." Well, as I've been saying throughout this whole book, your challenges are real, but it's your choice how you respond to them. Even if you need some adaptations, workarounds, or another person's support, there's probably *something* creative you can find to do.

As for creativity, talent is beside the point. This is for *you*, not for a museum or gallery. Try to do one creative act—be it doodling, humming a tune, cooking a nice dinner, baking bread, arranging a vase of flowers, making up a story, or writing a Haiku. It's all creative expression. Look to art as your healthy escape. Make your life a work of art.

For me, during the most debilitating part of convalescence, creativity took two forms: daily journaling and a project I named *Dream Blossoms: Dreams Blossom*, which I'll describe below.

Healing Words

Ever since I was a young girl, I've kept a journal to write my contemplations. I like writing longhand—the tactile, sensual act of pen caressing paper, the shape of words, thoughts flying across the page. But after my disc ruptured, when I was lying flat on my back, it was less painful for me to write daily journal bits on my laptop.

I knew I needed to write about what I was experiencing—for my sanity more than anything. Writing was cathartic. It gave me hope. Through it, I realized I have a lot to live for.

Writing can be a crucible for contemplation and alchemy, enabling you to dig deep and

- process emotions
- temporarily distract yourself from pain, suffering, fears, and worry
- record observations, chart progress over time, and make course corrections
- gain clarity and observe insights
- find nuggets of wisdom

What's more, research suggests "expressive writing may also offer physical benefits to people battling terminal or life-threatening diseases. . . . Writing about emotions and stress can boost immune functioning in patients with such illnesses as HIV/AIDS, asthma and arthritis."[86]

I encourage you to write about your healing crisis if you haven't already. Your writing needn't be perfect. You don't have to share it with others. It's powerfully healing.

Dream Blossoms: Dreams Blossom

After more than a year of being trapped in my disabled body—flat on my back, bedridden with the excruciating ruptured disc—I was strong enough to pick up my camera for the first time. It was only for five minutes, and definitely not while standing. I was elated—but the fact remained that I still couldn't physically *go* anywhere to take photographs.

One evening, on his way home from teaching, my husband bought me a bouquet of coral-colored roses. Recognizing I couldn't hold the camera for long, he fetched my dusty tripod, brought it to our bedroom, mounted my camera on it so as not to stress my fragile back, and placed the blossoms on a nearby dresser.

I mustered every ounce of strength, gritted my teeth against the pain, and began to shoot them. I found I could stand up for five minutes before the searing pain dialed up and sent me back to bed in tears. These brief moments weren't adequate to precisely compose my shots, but they opened a door to experimenting with close-up, soft-focus abstract images. It was a happy accident (check it out on this book cover!).

I've been taking photos of flowers since I was fifteen years old, but never with the passion, intensity, and inspiration of continual discovery I found in exploring the world of blossoms this way!

So the adventure began. After more than a year of deep suffering, I was beginning to see a wee bit of light, a bit of my old self—the artist—returning. My dreams began to blossom via exploration of those dreamy blossoms, hence the name *Dream Blossoms: Dreams Blossom*. I like the play on words to describe the dreamy quality of soft exposure photographs juxtaposed with my dreams blossoming into full bloom.

I didn't set out to create great art or a new body of work for a gallery show. It was all about rekindling passion . . . finding all the beauty I could express in that moment. It happened to be a dreary winter day, another day spent in bed, yet I discovered beauty.[87]

Art is healing expression and transformation—and creative play is a way to recharge, recover, and heal.

Like the healing process itself, *Dream Blossoms: Dreams Blossom* was born in baby steps—one or two photographs every week or two. I relished those brief moments of actual photography. In between sessions, I daydreamed about new flowers and colors to explore over the next few months. I leaned into the peace and beauty of their vibrant colors and sensuous curves. It gave me hope. As the series developed, my intention became this: *May these contemplative, atmospheric images help every heart find peace, healing, and joy.*

It's been nearly five years since the ruptured disc, and I still cannot hold my camera because of my spine's instability. But that's what tripods are for.

EXERCISE: CREATE SOMETHING, ANYTHING

It doesn't matter whether you believe you have artistic talent or not. You indeed have everything it takes to do expressive art. Follow the thread of inspiration wherever it leads you. Just play. There is no right or wrong way to do it. It needn't be beautiful. A perceived "mistake" can take you to a delicious landscape that wasn't on your map. That's the gift of creativity. The only thing that matters is your true expression. That, my friend, will heal you.

> Do not fear mistakes. There are none.
> —Miles Davis

Try anything and everything that lights you up:

- Crayons, watercolors, clay, colored pencils, acrylic paints, beading, mosaics, and other visual arts are all healing and fun. Remember what fun your first box of crayons was?

- Cook a nutritious meal. Create a colorful salad. Bake bread. That's creative expression too!

- Knit, sew, or embroider.
- Dance or do yoga.
- Design a garden or home improvement project.
- Music is hugely healing. It soothes the savage beast and helps our plants flourish. Play (or learn) an instrument, beat drums, shake rattles, or sound Tibetan bowls. Sing to the trees, hum, or chant.
- Creative writing, poetry, or journaling is highly therapeutic, as mentioned above.

If you wish for guidance, find a teacher.[88] Art transforms our emotions through expression. It helps heal trauma, as research demonstrates. When engaged in the arts, we can authentically express ourselves, reduce stress, and give voice to our fears, hopes, and dreams. Have fun!

> There is a vitality, a life-force, an energy, a quickening that is translated through you into action and because there is only one of you in all of time, this expression is unique. And if you block it, it will never exist through any other medium and be lost.
> —Martha Graham

31

PRACTICING PEACE

> If I could not be peaceful in the midst of danger, then the kind of peace I might have in simpler times is meaningless. If I could not find peace in the midst of difficulty, I knew I would never know real peace.
>
> —Thich Nhat Hanh, *At Home in the World*

Decades ago, I wrote a reminder on our kitchen chalkboard:

Go where the peace is . . .

A critically important key to navigating the roller coaster healing journey is finding deep peace. Peace assuages our feelings of loss, suffering, rootlessness, and deep sorrow.

Yet peace can be quite elusive in our busy, super-stressful, overstimulated world. Kids, family, job, finances, not to mention the state of the world . . . we've all got stress, and studies prove beyond a doubt that stress causes *dis-ease*,[89] the lack of ease and comfort which leads to disease.

Stress—and its mates worry, fear, rumination, frustration, anger, and overwhelm—does more than cause an unhealthy surge of cortisol to the bloodstream and trigger symptoms. *Stress steals this moment's peace.* Likewise, when we worry about tomorrow, we're stealing today's peace.

You can do all the right self-care stuff, but if you're living with chronic stress and don't *go where the peace is,* your body's ability to heal is hindered.

Minimizing Stress

We can find peace in more natural antidotes than tranquilizers:

- Controlling your reaction to stressors is all we *can* control. We can manage our response by shifting focus: try taking an aerial view of your life. *A year from now, will it have been worth the stress response?*

- Navigate away from the landmines that trigger your stress response (be they people, circumstances, work projects, or deadlines).

- Live mindfully in the present moment.

- Use essential oils, supplements, calming teas.

- Create a tranquil space.

- Infuse your day with mantras and meditations, worry beads/stones, Guatemalan worry dolls, crystals, etc. They've been used for centuries and are found worldwide today.

If you could adopt some of these proven ways to calm the ill effects of stress and prevent disease, why wouldn't you?

Exercise: Peace Power Breaks

When we can't avoid stressors completely, we can add a buffer zone. Think you're too busy to find peace in your day? It needn't be a large block. Find a minute (or five) stolen here and there between work projects, phone calls, or your daily duties.

I call these "Peace Power Breaks." Power Breaking is like power walking only it's the opposite of doing—it's *being*. There's peace in living with awareness in the present moment and focusing on your breath. Stop multitasking, take a breath, and be fully present in the moment of talking on the phone, doing dishes, driving your car, etc. Be aware of the beauty in this moment; just breathe. It brings peace and can be energizing when you're weary. This simple meditation on the breath is a powerful reset. I aim for five minutes per hour between work projects.

If you're prone to ruminate or catastrophize, simply recognize that, name it what it is (usually fear), then visualize the opposite. Here's an example: when I turned twenty-one, I was told I'd be wheelchair-bound by my mid-thirties. Whenever I began riffing on possible catastrophes, I'd put on music, and in my mind's eye, I choreographed myself dancing to it. Or I imagined sprouting wings and soaring through the air for a bird's-eye view of my favorite destinations. Or ice skating. Or gymnastics like Cirque du Soleil. "The Guided Journey" and "Day Tripping" chapters offer practices to put the brakes on rumination and lighten the spirit.

His Holiness the Dalai Lama has wise words for how we can find peace: "The most important factor in maintaining peace within oneself, in the face of any difficulty, is one's mental attitude. If it is distorted by such feelings as anger, attachment or jealousy, then even the most comfortable environment will bring one no peace. On the other hand, if one's attitude is generally calm and gentle, then even a hostile environment will have little effect on one's own mental peace. Since the basic source of peace and happiness is one's own mental attitude, it is worthwhile adopting means to develop it in a positive way."[90]

At the height of the pandemic, I emailed a friend:

Ken and I are finding peace in spite of this craziest of times. At night we read poetry together, watch movies, read books by a roaring fire. As I sit here, working a zillion hours, I'm able to look out the bedroom windows on blue sky and green trees . . . and breathe. In this moment, my life is perfect. We're healthy; we have everything we need. While the rest of the world is suffering miserably, we have this little safe haven of peace. I'm trying to hold onto that and be grateful for every peaceful moment.

Do I still have times of screaming pain? Yep. Tears of frustration and disappointment? You bet. Curse like a sailor from the pain? Hell, yes! Get snarky? Ask my husband. The point is, I quickly find my way back to a peaceful space.

We measure our pain on a scale of zero to ten. Do the same for peace. Where are you right now? An eight? Good. A two? Navigate your stressors and build in buffers of Peace Power Breaks to dial-up your peace index.

Deepening Peace?

How can we find pockets of deep peace amid the sea of suffering, pain, and loss and live in ease, grace, and flow? The prescription for healing is the peace found in silence—external, sure, but more importantly, inner silence. We must cultivate peace and harmony within ourselves. That doesn't mean we must live in a cave, on a mountaintop, or at an ashram. We find deep peace via:

- embracing acceptance, surrender, and letting go
- compassion for ourselves and others
- accepting imperfection and life's impermanence

While I cherish the wabi-sabi elements in my home—chippy paint on vintage furniture, a bowl of beach glass made soft from pummeling waves and sand—it has taken me a lifetime to embrace my own wabi-sabi-ness. With it comes deep peace.

Your Peace, World Peace

Peace for our world seems so out of reach, yet I've realized it's like the lyrics of that old song, "Let there be peace on earth, and let it begin with me." Peace, in fact, *does* begin with you and me making peace with our own healing journeys.

Our personal peace is a state of mind that permeates the sphere around us out into the world. Finding our peace is like a ripple in the pond of the planet. Just as a stone thrown into a pond creates concentric circles reaching out further and further, so too our peace ripples out into this world.

32

TALKING TO MYSELF: INTENTIONS

> Our intention creates our reality.
>
> —Dr. Wayne Dyer

In early 2016, I set a new intention: *Bring me the lessons I most need to learn to accelerate my spiritual growth.* Ha! I got a ruptured disc—which indeed taught me many lessons on my spiritual journey. It was a crash course (be careful what you wish for). Today I ask the lessons to come gently and less dramatically:

Bring me gentle lessons to help me achieve my highest purpose.

Words—spoken or thought—are magic. They change the vibration within and around you and rewire your brain. They can transform your life. Ultimately, it's not only what you do daily that heals you, but the intention set by you. The real alchemy comes when we brew words—intentions, affirmations, or mantras—with *belief.*

Exercise: Mantras and Affirmations

This tool is pretty straightforward. You begin by acknowledging and accepting your situation and then you speak true, positive, magic words to yourself.

For example, as you receive a healing procedure (be it acupuncture, massage, vaccination, or surgery)

- accept this healing
- visualize the positive outcome
- feel what it will be like when you're healed
- believe you are healing
- say your intention aloud or in your head:

I accept this medication/vaccine/treatment/procedure/surgery. I am so grateful for it. I am healing. So it is.

These favorites can bring a deep sense of safety and calm:

I am guided, protected, and healthy. Amen.

*

I accept this health crisis occurring in my life right now. I am grateful for the new opportunities it brings me.

*

*I love and bless the changes happening now.
I know I'm in the right place, at the right
time, doing the right thing
courageously with love, humor, and confidence.
All is well, and all will be well.*

Get more inspiration at SufferingtoThriving.com.

33
INNER SANCTUARY

It is not down in any map; true places never are.

—Herman Melville, *Moby Dick*

The healing journey can herald a time to migrate inward. As the outer landscape of our lives changes with illness, migrating inward can help us make sense of our world and reimagine a new way forward.

I call this the Inner Sanctuary. It's where you'll discover healing wisdom, authenticity, patience, peace, the strength to weather any storm, and spirituality (however you define it). They're all important to vibrant health. This doesn't prevent illness, of course, but it does help us navigate convalescence.

Whether you're in a claustrophobic MRI tube, enduring an uncomfortable procedure, in the hospital, or experiencing other stressors, you can always go to your Inner Sanctuary for tranquility and strength.

Magic and Its Benefits

> Spiritual practices give you the tools to deal with what life brings for you. . . . Your inner spirit has the strength to carry you through. The key is strengthening your connection with your inner spirit.
> —Sandra Ingerman, *Walking in Light*

The only sure thing is this present moment. It is a noble—and healing—goal, then, to fully embody this present moment with your full presence and mindfulness.

It's transformative to build a practice of active awareness into your life. The magic begins when we, in every moment of the day, are grounded in remembering the essence of who we are. We find it in our Inner Sanctuary.

Breaking the habit of mental chatter brings deep peace to your Inner Sanctuary. As you keep practicing, it becomes easier. I've been doing this for three decades and no longer have the monkey mind – that incessantly chattering inner voice – I once did. My habit is a centered, quiet mind, most of the time. It has accelerated my healing.

There's healing magic in this present moment, in stillness, a shift in perception. There's much research about how resting and doing nothing, even boredom,[91] can be quite healing. It's the perfect antidote for stress. Sure, we can purchase biofeedback devices and listen to stress-reducing podcasts. To *be* in your Inner Sanctuary, however, requires nothing more than your presence.

Ultimately, as your inner landscape changes, your outer world reflects it. For example, as your Inner Sanctuary becomes more tranquil, your life mirrors it—more peace, less drama.

Finding Your Inner Sanctuary

We have a tendency to think in terms of doing and not in terms of being. We think that when we are not doing anything, we are wasting our time. But that is not true. Our time is first

of all for us to be. To be what? To be alive, to be peaceful, to be joyful, to be loving. And that is what the world needs most.
—Thich Nhat Hanh

Your Inner Sanctuary is a *where* and a *when*. It's the place where you find awareness, mindfulness, and peace. It's when you can simply be and observe who you authentically are.

You'll find your Inner Sanctuary when you can sit in quiet stillness or contemplation without grasping onto the endless monkey mind chatter of your brain and without the constant distraction of the material world. It's what Frank MacEowen considers vital, "to find the sacred within life I must cultivate . . . sacred eyes."[92]

In this moment, just be. There, you'll experience the still point. A window of silence. A clearing of space and time where we go from inchoate ramblings to hearing whispers of future possibilities.

Be willing to say to your soul, "Show me the way." Then athletically listen, deeply with undivided attention, to your inner wisdom. Dive deep and listen to your heart's answer to the questions *What heals me? What is the true purpose of this illness/injury? What am I meant to learn? What is my true calling now?*

Exercise: Create Your Inner Sanctuary

Your Inner Healer will get you through your health crisis. Work daily to cultivate this strength by spending time in your Inner Sanctuary. It's as simple as finding moments of stillness to simply be.

- With awareness, savor the morsels of moments in your waking life.
- Sit in contemplation or visualization.
- Mindfully meditate, finding a style you enjoy.

- Just be. Thich Nhat Hahn teaches the practice of resting in the river[93] like a pebble, not going anywhere and not stressing about resting.

- If you find yourself resisting any of this, remember, what we resist identifies the work we need to do. *What we resist persists.*

With intention, everything is an opportunity for cultivating awareness, mindfulness, and healing: walking, bathing, washing dishes, lighting the fireplace, work, creativity.

If it's not already your practice, learn to meditate for healing. There are as many varieties of meditation as there are people. If stilling your mind hasn't worked for you, check out more active types of meditation ahead. You'll surely find one that resonates.

Try this practice for a month and see if you don't feel an improvement in your well-being. You might find it so enjoyable you'll make more time for it in your daily schedule.

> Beyond living and dreaming, there is
> something more important: Waking up.
> —Antonio Machado

Energy, light, and love . . . we sometimes look outside ourselves to find them. By cultivating our Inner Sanctuary, we discover they were here within us all along.

Be loyal and unwavering in your belief in your body's ability to heal. Its wisdom is within you. Find stillness and trust where the energies are pulling you.

Silence is the springboard for self-realization. Nature is a beautiful portal to silence.

> If you feel lost, disappointed, hesitant, or weak, return to yourself, to who you are, here and now, and when you get there, you will discover yourself, like a lotus flower in full bloom, even in a muddy pond, beautiful and strong.
> —Masaru Emoto, *Secret Life of Water*

34

YOU WILD THING

> Some days
> I am more wolf
> Than woman
> And I am still learning
> How to stop apologizing
> For my wild.
>
> —Nikita Gill, *Wild Embers*

Deep down, we're all wild animals inside. Human beings, yes, but Nature Beings, too.

Society beats the Nature Being out of us, scares us into the myth of separation, and tells us nature is a mighty enemy to be feared, the wilderness is something to be tamed and exploited, and animals are creatures to be controlled.

Yet we're all intrinsically part of nature. Whether you're aware of it or not, humans are interconnected with everything on the planet. We are of the same tribe. Look no further than the plight of the bees to become abundantly aware of just how interconnected we are.[94] If the recent pandemic and current climate crisis have taught us anything, it's that the health and well-being of every individual is inextricably linked to the health and well-being of all.

There's a fragile thread of connection running through the tapestry of the world, binding us to the planet, the land, animals, plants, and elements. Everywhere there are threads of connection weaving each of us and nature into One.

Why It Matters

> There is something infinitely healing
> in these repeated refrains of nature.
> —Rachel Carson

Nature knows how to heal. Over millions of years, our planet has recovered from epic cataclysms. Animals—from cats and dogs to the wild ones—innately know how to heal. So do we.

Mother Nature is literally our life support system. Everything we need—to heal what ails us, give us energy, restore our vitality—is found in nature.

What indigenous peoples around the globe know (and we are beginning to rediscover) is Mother Nature is a powerful healer and teacher. This idea is several centuries old, embedded in world religions and philosophies. For example, in the 1500s, Swiss physician, alchemist, theologian, philosopher Paracelsus believed all healing comes from nature. While I'm not saying a walk in the forest will cure your cancer, when you integrate nature's healing ways with Western and/or Eastern medicine, healing can be maximized.

Our ancestors lived close to the land—in balance and harmony with earth and in tempo with the seasons—and knew Mother Nature's healing ways. They lived in reciprocity with and respect for the land, its animals, and plants. As modern-day individuals, the more disconnected from nature we become, the sicker we get as individuals and as a species.

I'm not suggesting a return to the past but gleaning from it the knowledge that our health can improve when we get out into nature and truly connect with her. Some issues—like a bad mood or situational anxiety—can be completely reversed. For others—like chronic pain or depression—nature can help take the edge off and put things into perspective.

Researchers found that spending time in nature—even faux nature!—can lower blood pressure, promote cancer-fighting cells, improve well-being, and help with depression, anxiety, and ADHD.[95]

> The wilderness holds answers to questions
> man has not yet learned to ask.
> —Nancy Newhall

Broken Connection

Like plants and animals, we belong to this earth. Yet in our technology-based society, we've lost the essential connection today's indigenous cultures have to the land, earth, and all living things.[96]

Of earth's 8.7 million species, *Homo sapiens* is the only one so profoundly disconnected from Mother Earth. The EPA estimates that "Americans, on average, spend approximately 90 percent of their time indoors."[97] In the house or office, we observe nature from a window—or perhaps you see an urban jungle. Herein lies the root of our problems, from environmental degradation and man-made climate change to our own declining health: most humans choose to live divorced from nature.

Ecology professor Robin Wall Kimmerer asked her students to rate the negative interactions between humans and nature. She was shocked when "nearly every one of the two hundred students said confidently that humans and nature are a bad mix. These were third-year students who had selected a career in environmental protection." In a later survey on positive interactions, "The median response was 'none.'"[98]

What's needed to heal ourselves and our planet is to enjoy more fresh air and sunshine wherever we can find it. We must recover—individually and as a community—our connection with nature.

> This is what is the matter with us. We are bleeding at the
> roots, because we are cut off from the earth and sun and stars,
> and love is a grinning mockery, because, poor blossom,
> we plucked it from its stem on the tree of Life, and
> expected it to keep on blooming in our
> civilized vase on the table.
> —D.H. Lawrence

LEARNING TO RECONNECT

> When despair for the world grows in me
> and I wake in the night at the least sound
> in fear of what my life and my children's lives may be,
> I go and lie down where the wood drake
> rests in his beauty on the water, and the great heron feeds.
> I come into the peace of wild things . . .
> I rest in the grace of the world, and am free.
> —Wendell Berry, "The Peace of Wild Things"

For centuries, civilizations the world over have found spending time in nature to be deeply healing. Modern-day indigenous cultures also believe in restoring the body and soul through connection with nature. The Japanese practice of *shinrin-yoku* ("forest bathing")—taking long walks in the woods to reconnect with nature and fortify health—has been found to reduce stress, anxiety, depression, and anger; strengthen the immune system; improve cardiovascular and metabolic health; and boost overall well-being.[99]

On a lovely spring day, you pick a handful of wildflowers—and see how quickly they wilt. Severed from their source, Mother Nature's nutritious earth, they wither and die. They cannot survive. Neither can we.

I'm in nature nearly every day, but on the rare occasions I can't find time, I'm a lot like those wilting wildflowers. I'm what you'd call a nature girl and a nemophilist (a lover of woods and forests), so nature is my "go-to" when I need stress relief and/or healing. I've learned a lifetime of healing lessons from Gaia herself:

- the patience of plants and animals as they live in harmony with the seasons
- their ability to heal themselves
- how they take only what they need
- how the planet is our best and only life support system capable of providing everything we need to thrive
- the interconnectedness of everything

In the last chapter, we discussed how inner peace helps shape our health. Fortunately, you don't need to move to a remote mountaintop or hidden forest. Inner peace can easily be cultivated by being in nature—anywhere you can find it. Even in cities, you can tap into nature: a park, a lone tree against which to sit, the sky full of clouds.

It's about getting back in sync with Mother Earth. If you don't have a connection with nature, you must learn to belong to the land where you live, the community of plants and animals, and the planet.

Exercise: Syncing with Nature

- Commit to spending time out-of-doors getting to know plants and animals, the geography of the landscape, its ancestral inhabitants, and the elements. It doesn't matter where: in your backyard hammock, a city park, wildlife preserve, national park, botanical garden, beach, desert, farmland, or someplace more exotic. If there's water nearby, so much the better. Water's negative ions have healing power. If you're bedridden, pull back the curtains, open the window, and rest your gaze on the trees and landscape. If you have no natural vista, look up at the sky and find some peace there.

- Go into nature with a sense of reverence and a curious spirit about her wonders. Keep an open mind and heart. We are all part of this living, breathing world, woven into this web of life. *How can you reconnect with that? How can you make time to commune with nature? What can plants, animals, and the land teach you? What are the threads of connection between us?*

- What do you do once you're in nature? Simply be. Do nothing. Place your awareness on what is. Take off your shoes and absorb the good earth energy through the soles of your feet. It's called earthing.[100] Our lives become richer as we slow down and, with pure awareness, spend time in the natural world. No multitasking. No devices. Not even reading. I don't need to tell you the fast pace of our modern world is causing us all stress and—if severe and sustained—even trauma. Nature meditation is a refreshing and restorative way to clear the mind and relax the body.

- Find beauty in everything. Even the dandelion pushing up through the concrete. Admire its strength and tenacity. Its seeds will take flight and travel on the wind beyond its city sidewalk.

- Be a mindful observer but also know you're part of this living environment, as essential as a bird, a tree, or the landscape.

- Express gratitude to strengthen your communion with Mother Earth. Recognize she's our life support system; send her love. When you're out in nature—

even if it's your backyard garden or local park—gift her seeds, water, flower petals, tobacco, sage, nuts, or oatmeal for the critters; hum to the trees; sing with the birds. Above all, give her the greatest gift: your mindful attention. When we pay attention, we understand nature is always speaking to us in signs, symbols, and messages.

- Learn to live in harmony with the cycles of the sun, moon, tides, four seasons, and the elements. For instance, with the availability of foods year-round, we've forgotten how to eat with the seasons, that is, to only eat fruits and veggies when they are in season locally. The bigger lessons of living by the seasons include resting and going inward in winter, planting seeds of intention and creativity that bloom in the spring, coming to full bloom in summer, and reaping the harvest of our actions in the fall. This alignment is doubly important if you live in an urban environment.

Live in each season as it passes; breathe the air, drink the drink, taste the fruit, and resign yourself to the influences of each.
—Henry David Thoreau

For better physical and mental health, our lives must be more in sync with nature—more like the universe (expanding/contracting), the moon (new beginnings / waxing to completion), the tides (ebbing/flowing), breathing (inhaling/exhaling), the seasons (resting in fall and winter / growing in spring and summer)—instead of full-on summer, high tide, full moon, and expansion all the time. Once I fell into step with the flow of nature, I began to recover my health. By deepening your roots into Mother Earth, you too will find powerful healing.

Nature can be a constant source of peace, wonder, and inspiration.

When we're under the weather or down for the count, it's hard to physically *get* to nature—and easy to become out of sync with her cycles. When convalescing and shut in, I gazed out our bedroom windows at trees and sky and the dreamy passing clouds, listened to birdsong and thunderstorms, and reveled in the scent of rain or freshly fallen snow. These experiences grounded me, connected me to Source, and were vital to my healing. Even connecting with nature through the window brings, as Wendell Berry said, "the peace of wild things."[101]

Healing the Planet

Our planet is in peril, and what's required to save it is nothing short of our own reconnection with nature and living in right alignment. Humans take—oxygen, food, minerals, resources—rape the land, and kill off animals to the brink of earth's sixth mass extinction.

When we don't honor Mother Nature's call, she gets louder and louder. Global climate change is a good example of this: catastrophic hurricanes and wildfires—decades before they were predicted to manifest this direly. It's the eleventh hour. We urgently need to reconnect, for our planet's survival is hanging in the balance. Many wonderful organizations share ways to help.[102]

Individually and collectively, we must heal our relationship with Gaia. Each of us can make a difference by living in harmony with nature, with reciprocity, in a sustainable manner. In turn, we'll live our own lives in better health and leave a healthier planet for future generations.

35

DAY TRIPPING: DON'T GIVE UP YOUR DREAMS

> Reach high, for stars lie hidden in you.
> Dream deep, for every dream precedes the goal.
>
> —Rabindranath Tagore

Here's an excerpt from one of my journal entries:

December 28, 2016—*I wish I were well and in Paris or Venice now. In my mind, in flights of fancy, I'm there. Or the Scottish Highlands, Martinique, Hawai'i, the Greek Islands—retracing memories of more healthy, carefree times. It was all so different then. Life somehow was lighter, easier, more elegant. I may never get it back—but I'll always have memories and daydreams.*

As kids in school, we aren't encouraged to daydream. As we grow up, it becomes clear society devalues daydreams—and nightdreams—as make-believe, worthless, "only a dream." Yet ancient cultures—especially the Greeks, Norsemen, shamanic healers, indigenous cultures of the Americas, Celtic druids, and Aboriginal Australians—actively sought healing wisdom from dreams and vision quests.[103]

Daydreams and nightdreams are sacred guidance from your embodied wisdom. We are dreaming our world into being, co-creating reality. As far back as Plato and Aristotle and more recently with Carl Jung, James Hillman, Robert Moss, Dr. Stephen Aizenstat, and other wise minds, it has been believed that our dreams are "a little hidden door in the innermost and most secret recesses of the soul."[104] They shape the energy of our world. Moss and Aizenstat tell us that *dreams are medicine.*

Dreaming Your New Life

We daydream all day long. *Why not be intentional and daydream new possibilities and opportunities, a new way of being?* Imagination is your most powerful tool. What we can imagine, we can become. Dreaming is the path.

> The stronger the imagination is, the less it is merely imaginary and the more is it in harmony with truth.
> —Rabindranath Tagore

Nowhere is this more potent and potentially transformative than when we're convalescing. Imaginative daydreams and nightdreams can be healing and potent soul work. Plus they can help us cope with feeling otherwise left out of "real life" because of our malady.

Never doubt your capacity to dream a better life. Escape from reality is sometimes vital to get through a difficult time. To give up daydreaming is to give up hope. Don't give up your dreams—they are your wishes on wings.

If you want to change your life, change your daydreams. Yes, you can daydream your new life into existence by envisioning a better moment. Instead of focusing on your disease, focus on dream-shaping your new world.

> Throw your dream into space like a kite, and you do not know what it will bring back, a new life, a new friend, a new love, a new country.
> —Anaïs Nin

Exercise: Daydream Play Date

- Make a date with yourself for the sole purpose of daydreaming. Enter it on your calendar, be it fifteen minutes or an hour. Look forward to it with anticipation as you would a date with a loved one.

- Over the next few days, set an intention to daydream about something exciting, journey to someplace new or to bring back wisdom.

- When the date arrives, unplug devices. Create a sacred space by lighting a candle or incense, making a cup of tea, or whatever ritual signals something important is about to occur.

- Get comfortable in a place where you're safe and undisturbed to journey. Close your eyes, breathe a few deep breaths, and relax your body.

- In your mind's eye, find your favorite spot of solitude: a serene beach, woods, etc. Imagine it vividly. *What scents? Sounds? Is there music? What season is it? What are you wearing? What are you doing?* The more vividly you imagine it, the more empowering the experience will be. Give yourself time to explore what makes you happy.

- Now imagine a tether holding your spirit to your body. Gently untie the bow. Allow yourself to fly free, dance, swim—whatever tickles your fancy. Enthusiastically feel this sensation, the freedom, the joy.

- Take time to enjoy your imagination and explore this inner world. Meet up with the dog of your dreams, tango with an exciting partner, ride a beautiful horse across the prairie, or slalom down a fast slope of powder. Sprout wings and feel the breeze lift you higher, leaving your body a little speck in the distance. The point is to take your mind off your physical/mental issues and just enjoy being *you*.

Another adventure is to daydream about a new project idea, the solution to a challenge, or a new life. There's a whole world of possibilities and opportunities here. Be open to the magic and enchantment. Be open to hearing your intuition, your Inner Healer, your inner dreamer.

How do you feel afterward? What would you like to explore next time? Did you receive any messages of inner wisdom? Ideas for what you need more of in your life? Less of? Write about it in your journal. There's alchemy in your words.

I realize it sounds simplistic, but it works. I daydreamed my own business into being as well as new creative paintings, poems, and photographic series.

> You were born with ideals and dreams.
> You were born with greatness.
> You were born with wings.
> You are not meant for crawling, so don't.
> You have wings.
> Learn to use them and fly.
> —Rumi

Exercise: Nightdreams

For centuries, cultures around the globe have sought out dreams for healing. All dreams come to help us heal—physically, mentally, or spiritually. Nightdreams can warn us of a condition, show the root cause of disease, suggest a remedy, urge us to rest, and give us guidance. I've had some tremendously powerful dreams that have guided me to heal conditions and life issues.

Our minds bestow healing dreams from deep within the subconscious. We can enhance this by setting an intention. After your evening meditation or gratitude practice, as you lie down, ask for a healing dream. Passionflower, blue lotus, and mugwort teas may enhance nightdreams, and relaxation too. Say,

Tonight I intend to receive a healing dream.
Show me how to heal my body and mind, what I need to grow.
Point the way forward. I'm grateful for this healing.

Be sure to record your daydreams/nightdreams, their healing messages, and their meanings in a *Book of Dreams* journal.[105]

> Some day you will be old enough to
> start reading fairy tales again.
> —C.S. Lewis

In deciphering your dreams, explore the archetypes of myths, folk tales, fairy tales, and fables.[106] Your healing journey and the clues for navigating your road to transformation—it's all there. For centuries these stories have been shared from generation to generation because, well, there are no new stories—only variations of the themes of the existing archetypes. You may feel you're alone in your experience. But since the beginning of time, your story, your search for a way through the darkness, your quest for meaning . . . it's all been told before, through the archetypes, for the purpose of learning.

These stories, as old as time, remind us that our new lives begin at the end of our comfort zones. They teach of dying to be reborn, shape-shifting to overcome adversity, sacrificing something that no longer serves to make space so something new can emerge, and being stripped bare to see what remains of ourselves. For example, your healing journey may have stripped you of nearly everything that was once your "normal" life. *What*

remains of you? What matters most? What are you passionate about? What are your gifts? How can you use them to heal?
   Your daydreams and nightdreams will help you heal.

> Everything we formulate in the imagination, if we formulate
> it strongly enough, realizes itself in the circumstances
> of our life, acting either through our own souls,
> or through the spirits of nature.
> —William Butler Yeats

36

THE GUIDED JOURNEY: VISUALIZATION & MEDITATION

> You are part of the Eternal Life. Awaken and expand your consciousness in God so that your concept of yourself ceases to be limited to the little body.
>
> —Paramahansa Yogananda

Your mind is immensely powerful. As we explored in "Change Your Mind," the mind can help you heal, visualize a new dream for your life, and take you to a better place when you're experiencing something painful or traumatic. Research demonstrates that guided imagery and visualization can have a profound beneficial effect on our health. Imagery has been found "to stimulate our immune systems, to increase or decrease blood flow to areas of the body, and thus to influence healing."[107]

Visualizations and meditations are not quick-fix pills. Clear intention, belief, and regular practice are key to making these tools work for you.

Prior to getting into the visualizations and meditations, here is a word about three important building blocks:

- breathwork
- body scan
- grounding and centering

BREATHWORK

Breath is life. For thousands of years, across many cultures, breathwork has been a foundation of healing. Throughout the day, your breathing is somewhat shallow. Yet a deep, conscious breath is an anchor, bringing nourishing oxygen through your blood and cells that can accelerate healing, reduce discomfort, and lower inflammation—and consequently, pain. Another benefit is deep relaxation, which works to combat the damaging effects of stress.

> The breath is the ultimate tool. Go into the breath. Exhale and accept the gift that the universe is giving you with every inhalation.
> —Mary Burmeister, *The Touch of Healing*

One conscious breath is better than hundreds of regular breaths. My practice is to take three deep healing breaths every hour, at least. Commit to this, and you'll see better overall health and stress relief.

Every meditation below begins with taking three or more deep cleansing breaths. Here's a simple yet powerful healing breath practice:

- Get comfortable, relax your body, and steady your breathing.

- Set an intention that your breaths will bring you energy and healing.

- Exhale fully. This is key because you cannot inhale fully unless you first fully exhale.

- Breathe in slowly and steadily, filling your lungs deeply.

- Visualize white or golden light entering every cell of your body.

- Hold your breath gently for three seconds, visualizing the light-filled oxygen flowing through your entire body, circulating around any sick/injured parts.

- Release the breath slowly and fully, visualizing the exhaled breath as grey fog carrying disease or pain.

- Between breaths, feel your aliveness in this present moment. Enjoy the now. Smile. If thoughts of the future/past enter your mind, simply observe them and return to the breath.

- Repeat this inhale/exhale several times: inhale peace, love, and joy, envisioning them permeating your body. Then exhale peace, love, and joy to every sentient being. On the last exhale, give thanks for the healing.

Repeat the steps above throughout your day as needed, especially upon waking and before sleep, and when stressed or in discomfort. It's subtle but transformative!

> Breathe deeply, until sweet air extinguishes the burn of fear in your lungs and every breath is a beautiful refusal to become anything less than infinite.
> —D. Antoinette Foy

Body Scan

The body scan is mindfully tuning in to your body and noticing pain and tension. While it has numerous benefits in itself, from relaxation to sleep,[108] it's also an excellent prelude to meditation. Here's how to do it:

- Take three deep cleansing breaths. With each breath, relax your face, eyes, eyebrows, scalp, ears, neck, and shoulders. Let a wave of relaxation ripple down your entire body.

- Focus on each point in your body—from feet to head (if you wish to lift your energy), or from head to feet (for grounding) —mindful of each muscle, each body part. For example, focus on your feet; breathe golden or white light into them. Visualize this light growing stronger and brighter through every cell in your body up to your head. See it illuminate the unwell parts.

- *Where is the tension? Pain? Where do you feel energy depleted?* Breathe into them.

- Exhale, envisioning grey fog that carries with it any illness, pain, infection, loss, injury, or fatigue.

- Now focus on body parts that are not experiencing discomfort and notice what it feels like to be in perfect health. Say thank you to each pain-free, disease-free area.

- Turn to the place(s) where you're experiencing a health challenge. This may be a single point or a vast area enduring a storm of nerve pain, muscle pain, or extreme fatigue. Imagine a current of golden healing light pouring in from above and focusing on the affected areas. If you suffer from fatigue, send energy through your entire being. Draw in this energy simply by breathing. Exhale any pain, infection, fatigue, or disease. Do this for as long as you need.

- When you're ready to come back to your awareness, imagine a cocoon of healing light or bubble of protection surrounding you.

- Give thanks for the healing. When you're ready, open your eyes.

How do you feel? If this was helpful, you might wish to incorporate it into your daily activities or Monk Morning. If this particular body scan didn't work for you, many free resources are available online.

Grounding and Centering

Whether you've just woken up from a nightmare or are having difficulty falling asleep, when you're awake but feeling spacey and unable to focus, or if you're having trouble coming back down to earth following a meditation, visualization, or daydream, grounding and centering brings you back to the present moment. It can calm you before a speech or social encounter, during/after an argument, or when you're feeling weak, vulnerable, stressed, or unsafe. It's also important before visualization or meditation.

- First, get comfortable in your chair and plant both feet flat. Take a few cleansing breaths, filling your lungs and abdomen, relaxing your body from your scalp to your toes, feeling your body settle in and get heavier as you relax.

- Now imagine roots sprouting from inside your abdomen and spreading downward with each breath, down through your root chakra, down your legs, out through the soles of your feet, and through the floor, putting deep roots into the soft warm earth, communing with tree roots, crystals, and rich earth.

- Feel the earth's energy travel up your "roots" into your body, slowly spreading through every cell to the top of your head. From your crown chakra, the energy sprinkles up and out like a fountain, falling all around you like a bubble of energy before returning back to the earth.

- Keep running your energy this way: pulling energy up from the ground, through your body, out your crown chakra, all around you, and repeat.

- Continue as long as needed. You are grounded, strong, and stepping into your power. Bask in this feeling, letting it permeate your being.

- Notice this feeling aggregating in your abdominal area (solar plexus) as your energy begins to center itself there. Feel the balance, calm, and strength. You're centered.

- When you're ready to come back to your regular life, watch the roots gently absorb into the ground and take three deep breaths. Open your eyes, stretch, and go about your day centered and grounded in your body.

You can come back to this place whenever needed. Hold a crystal for a deeper experience.

VISUALIZATION

Now that you have the basic tools of breathwork, body scan, grounding, and centering under your belt, let's discuss visualization.

What we think about, we bring about. For decades, elite athletes have been employing visualized imagery to achieve peak performance.[109] Research tells us that thinking about an activity stimulates the brain, nerves, and muscles, simulating the actual activity. "When athletes visualize or imagine a successful competition, they actually stimulate the same brain regions as you do when you physically perform that same action. Visualization in sports or mental imagery is a way of conditioning for your brain for successful outcomes."[110]

What's more, studies have shown that simply imagining the immune system working has a significant effect on T cells. Our brains don't distinguish between imagination and reality. It's why visualization is a powerful tool for dreaming things into reality.

I practice visualization daily—picturing success for the day ahead, an increase in the number of steps I can walk, or a positive outcome in a vexing health or life situation. Below are some of my favorite visualizations, but once you get the hang of it, create your own. The sky's the limit.

To achieve the best results, use all your senses. Also, personalize your visualizations. For example, my friend uses a visualization below but imagines the iconic Pac-Man character (from the old video game) eating away cancer cells in her body. Recently she was told her cancer is in remission without chemo or radiation.

> Imagination is better than a sharp instrument.
> To pay attention, this is our endless proper work.
> —Mary Oliver, "Yes! No!"

MEDITATION

Many people believe they "fail" at meditation as they are unable to empty their minds of chatter. There are many ways to meditate besides trying to empty your mind of thought. Experiment to find what works for you. For example, notice with mindful awareness the thoughts or worries that stream through your mind. *Ah yes, there's something I'm worried about, there's an item for the to-do list*, etc. Pay attention to how your mind works—even fifteen minutes a day is valuable. Another way is to follow a guided imagery meditation. Or focus mindfully on the breath, finding stillness in the place between inhaling and exhaling. Find a meditation practice that works for you.

Through meditation we shift to a higher consciousness of mindful awareness, inner peace, and well-being. Meditation enables us to find a place of limitless potential. We are not our ailing bodies but infinite spirits who can live in peace and joy despite our health (or any other) crisis.

As with so many traditional approaches, meditation is beginning to find support among Western scientists. Leonard Calabrese writes, "Mind-body interventions like meditation and mindfulness have been gaining empirical support for their ability to lessen perceived stress, alleviate depression, reduce loneliness, downregulate central inflammatory pathways, and benefit immune regulation. This may be beneficial for people suffering from chronic inflammatory conditions such as rheumatoid arthritis, inflammatory bowel disease, and asthma, in which psychological stress plays a role."[111]

There's also research on the health benefits of group drumming, among other things.[112]

We meditate in order to quiet the mind, to stop the chatter (monkey mind), to make space for new insights, for creativity to happen, and to allow intuition and our Inner Healer to speak. With practice, we can learn to quiet the mind most of the time. It becomes a habit if we cultivate it. I practice intentional non-thinking, and breaking negative thought patterns before they get hooked. As a result, I've developed a mostly quiet mind by choosing an intentional path.

Some people (myself included) find holding a crystal in their hand takes meditation up a notch. Stones can bring clarity and healing, and through your meditation, you're infusing the crystal with talismanic power. For an extra feeling of protection, begin your visualization or meditation by imagining yourself inside a quartz crystal. Experiment with specific crystals' properties and determine which are best for your meditations.

Micro-Disciplines

Short on time? Micro-disciplines to the rescue! Even short bursts of these tools can yield big results. Mindfulness micro-discipline is a great strategy when you're in queue at the post office or grocery store, stuck in traffic, cooking, showering, waiting for a Zoom meeting to begin, or enduring a medical procedure. Instead of becoming impatient, agitated, and checking the time, you can:

- breathe deep and tap into how you're feeling physically and emotionally
- breathe in peace and breathe out love—to yourself, your medical team, friends, family, community, Mother Earth, and/or all sentient beings
- say a quiet affirmation, mantra, prayer, or word of gratitude
- envision a place of beauty that deeply resonates with you
- practice a variation on awareness meditation: observe details surrounding you (light, sounds, colors, scents)

You'll find that time spent waiting can be a gift.

But micro-disciplines aren't limited to waiting around. Try applying the examples above to an active meditation:

- walking meditation
- dancing, movement, or drumming meditation
- drawing or painting meditation

The physical, emotional, and mental benefits are enormous. What started for me as a few stolen minutes here and there a couple of decades ago has grown into a practice of mindful awareness woven into every day: living in the present moment.

Your Toolkit of Visualizations and Meditations

Now let's get started with my three favorite visualizations and meditations (you'll find more at SufferingtoThriving.com). Remember, for the deepest and most relaxing healing experience, be sure to start with breathwork, a body scan, and grounding and centering.

After you've finished, take a moment to reflect on your experience and journal your insights. If nothing came to you, try again tomorrow.

Your Personal Power Spot
In your mind's eye, imagine a place that speaks to you. It could be somewhere you've lived or visited, a pilgrimage you'd like to make, or someplace found in the imaginal realm. It could be a beach, park, mountain vista, or a garden—somewhere you feel energized, invigorated, peaceful, content, safe, strong, comfortable, or connected to something infinite. *Feeling* the energy is an essential part of the magic. This is your power place, your spiritual home.

You can come here any time you need to listen to your inner guidance, feel safe, or find solace from discomfort. You might find more than one location speaks to you. That's fine. In fact, I have a few personal power spots: a sacred place in the high desert of New Mexico, a mystic loch in the Scottish Highlands, azure waters of the Lesser Antilles where I first swam with dolphins, and a jungle temple in the Yucatan.

There's no right or wrong place. Wherever you feel pulled to be, this is your power spot.

Explore this place and its surrounding area. Use all your senses and tap into your emotions. In this spot, you're in perfect health. *What does that look like? What does that feel like?* If you're physically challenged, perhaps you wish to imagine yourself running like a wolf does, swimming like a dolphin, or soaring like a bird (or a drone) for a bird's-eye perspective on your life or challenges. *What do you wish to discover? What problem do you wish to solve? As you explore your surroundings, do you receive any messages from your imagination? Images? Words? Symbols?*

The more you play with this, the more likely you'll begin to find healing messages from your subconscious.

This type of visualization has been particularly helpful to me in getting through the COVID-19 pandemic lockdowns, as well as when I was housebound and bedridden for years. I also use it every time I'm in the MRI tube.

The Cone of Protection
When you're feeling fear or anxiety and wish to create a safe space, this is a quick, easy visualization that can be done anywhere—in the car, at work, on a city street, in the middle of a jungle, before a medical procedure or surgery, or to ease your mind before slumber. Within seconds, you can surround yourself or your loved ones with protection. For example, every day I take a moment to create a bright white cone of protection for our forest.

Don't get hung up on the cone's shape or color. If a golden pyramid or a pink bubble feels right to you, visualize that. The emotion and belief you pour into the exercise are what matters most. It goes like this . . .

Visualize what you wish to protect. Imagine in your mind a ray of white light emanating from your index finger as you draw a circle on the ground around the area to be protected. Imagine the circle vibrating with light, which rises into the sky, converging in a point high above, creating a cone of protection, shimmering white.

Breath in the protective light. You are guarded and protected.

Finding Your Inner Healer Meditation
Where in your body is your healing wisdom or intuition? What does it look like? There's no right or wrong answer. Perhaps you'll find it in your heart, behind your third eye, or in your gut (the brain in your belly). Meditate on the question *Where is my healing wisdom located?* This helps you find your unique embodied intelligence.

Write or draw observations in your journal. Connect with your Inner Healer every day. It's like a muscle. Work it to make it stronger. Get creative and have some fun! Ask questions and be patient about receiving answers. Our Inner Healer doesn't always speak up loudly. Sometimes we need to take a journey to meet it where it resides and petition it to enlighten us.

37

GOOD VIBRATIONS

> We are slowed down sound and light waves, a walking bundle of frequencies tuned into the cosmos. We are souls dressed up in sacred biochemical garments and our bodies are the instruments through which our souls play their music.
>
> —Unknown

LIVING IN A VIBRATING WORLD

Everything in the universe is energy—atoms vibrating at a frequency ranging from low to high: trees, rocks, food, music, our planet, ourselves. Nothing in the universe is *not* vibrating. In scientific terms, our planet "behaves like a gigantic electric circuit. Its electromagnetic field surrounds and protects all living things with a natural frequency pulsation of 7.83 hertz on average. . . . Interestingly, 7.83 hertz is also the human brain's average alpha frequency."[113] We are energy beings, and the earth's vibration is healing.

Vibrational energy is invisible, but we can see evidence of it at work. Musicians witness this firsthand. In a gathering of stringed instruments, when one string is plucked, all the others vibrate too (without being touched). Same with drums—bang a drum and nearby drums will vibrate. Same with pendulum clocks. It's called *entrainment*. Research demonstrates that sound brings our brains into entrainment within four minutes.

Inanimate objects vibrate, but so do all living things. To demonstrate this, teachers have brought two living plants to their classrooms and labeled them "love" and "hate." Students are instructed to speak to one plant kindly with high-vibration words of love and admiration every day; to the other plant, they speak low-vibration, mean, hateful words. You can guess the outcome—the plant spoken to consistently with loving messages thrives while the other withers. Similarly, an internationally renowned scientist demonstrated how our thoughts, words, and feelings—loving or hateful—affect water molecules and snowflakes.[114]

How Vibrations Affect Humans

Great scientists and philosophers have agreed, everything is energy. You—your thoughts, moods, actions, words, attitude—have a vibrational frequency. Although it's invisible to the eye, it's perceptible to energy workers and healers. Perhaps you've felt it? Walk into a room of negative energy—a tense meeting, a place where something terrible happened—the bad vibes are palpable. If we stay in that environment, we'll notice our own vibration plummeting to match the surroundings.

Higher vibrations are discernable too. Play your favorite upbeat song, and your spirits lift. You'll feel it when you're around places and people who make you feel happy, or when you're in love, or when you feel deep gratitude, or when you're passionate about a project and "in the zone."

Research shows vibrational energy indeed affects our bodies and thoughts—which, according to physics, are mostly responsible for the reality we experience. In other words, vibrating at a low (negative) frequency attracts more of it to your life. Positive energy attracts more positive energy.

Here's why. You are composed of vibrating atoms of stardust and water—up to 60 percent of the adult body is water, and the brain and heart are 73 percent water.[115] It's well established that sound waves travel faster in water than air, so it makes sense that vibration permeates every cell of our bodies, and quickly.

Anything that isn't raising your vibrational energy is likely lowering it. Today we're bombarded with electromagnetic force (EMF) radiation from our devices, negative news, radiation from X-rays and MRIs, toxins in our environment and food, etc. Anytime we can counteract these bad vibrations with our positive vibrational tools, we help our bodies heal.

High vibrations cleanse negativity, invigorate life, and promote healing. When we begin to work intentionally with energy, dramatic healing can occur. Imagine how this practice could benefit your health, your home, your community, and our world!

Vibrational healing—a.k.a. energy medicine—is not a new concept. It dates back several thousand years (some say seventy thousand). It's a core practice of ancient Chinese and Japanese healers, India's Ayurvedic masters, Australian Aborigines, North/South American shamans, and medicine wo/men of indigenous cultures who've used energy medicine to heal body and mind.

This healing modality continues to be applied with positive outcomes in mainstream society today. Take drumming for example. Cultures the world over—ancient and present-day—employ drumming for healing, including drumming meditation.[116] Everyone can benefit from banging a drum, ringing a bell, or humming. *You don't need to be a musician to create and benefit from sound healing vibrations.*

Turns out that energy medicine is the future of healing. Doctors, hospitals, and hospice centers across the country and world have integrated energy medicine practices—Reiki for example—to benefit health.[117]

Raise Your Vibration

Your thoughts shape your vibrational energy field. The higher your vibration, the more quickly you can manifest health and other outcomes. Change your thoughts and where you put your attention, and you can create a new future. This is the law of attraction. It's physics.

No one can sustain a perfectly high vibration; we all vacillate between highs and lows. However, we can aim to raise our vibration incrementally throughout our days, by doing the following:

1) enlisting the help of an energy worker (who specializes in Reiki, crystal healing, scientifically-based sound healing, breathwork, Qigong, etc.) for energy balancing

2) working daily to maintain a higher vibration

3) keeping your vibrational and acoustic space clean

Let's unpack how you can raise your vibration:

- First, tune in to your vibration and be mindful of the vibrations around you. Pay attention to where in your body you feel the bad vibes: gut? shoulders? back? neck? heart? For me, bad vibes are dark clouds of tension, jangly nerves, tightness in my shoulders, or a snappish mood. Good vibes bring a feeling of euphoria and deep peace. *Where do you feel the vibes?*

- *Who, what, where, and when do you feel a higher vibration?* Make a list in your journal.

- Experiment with doing more of what makes your vibration higher and less of what doesn't. By cutting out low vibrations, you're raising your vibration.

- Live on purpose. Every day, set an intention to raise your frequency to be in harmony with who you intend to be. From the moment you wake until the moment you drift off to sleep, be intentional about your thoughts, speech, actions, attitude, and activities—

people you engage with, places you go, your food/drink, and entertainment. Curate each day by imbuing your environment with high vibrations through positive thoughts, words, and feelings. We're not talking about manufactured or fake positive thoughts. Instead, aim for heartfelt positive thoughts with passionate emotion behind them. Remember those classroom plants?

- As we've learned, gratitude, meditation, and visualization have high vibrations.

- Nature is high-vibration and healing. It's no accident we felt so alive and joyful as children playing outside.

- Hold a crystal, listen to Tibetan or crystal singing bowls, listen to or make uplifting music, bang a drum, sing or hum, or use tuning forks[118] as you visualize healing sound waves traveling through your body.[119]

Raise your vibe and you'll not only 1) feel good but you'll also 2) be a magnet who attracts more high-vibration people and circumstances and you'll 3) be in alignment with your most authentic self and your highest good.

Your journal can help you cultivate your vibrational awareness and curate choices that will ultimately lead to a higher vibe day—and life. Your list is a touchstone when you find yourself, as we all do, in a rough patch, a funky mood, or a negative place and need to hit the reset button. Observe your vibrations and those around you and make a different choice. We become the product of our choices.

There's a whole world of vibrational healing out there for you to explore:

- acupuncture, acupressure, Reiki, chakra work
- uplifting music and art
- crystal therapy

- humming and voice as a sonic healer, tuning forks, sound baths[120]
- plant medicine
- affirmations, mantras, positive thoughts, intentions, visualizations, meditation
- Yoga, Qigong, Tai Chi, EFT tapping

> If you want to find the secrets of the universe, think in terms of energy, frequency, and vibration.
> —Nikola Tesla

CRYSTALS

Every day I meditate with or wear a crystal to align with its highly refined, healing vibration. Crystals transmute heavy energy and cannot hold or transmit a negative vibration. It may sound woo-woo, but crystals—formed in the earth over more than ten million years—are known to science and technology as transducers that transform energy. They've been used for centuries by healers around the globe as well as modern-day Reiki masters.

I find crystals give a peaceful vibe conducive to healing. Whether you feel their energy magic in the form of positivity, healing, grounding, or protection—or whether you display them as a decoration or talisman in your home to imbue peaceful vibes—why not give them a try?

At any time in your day, you can ask, *What's my vibration right now? High? Low? What's my intention for raising my vibrational energy?* Make a go-to list of energy lifters to infuse your day with high vibrations.

> There is no healing journey without the vibrational frequency of love.
> —Jeralyn Glass

38

BON VOYAGE

> The book doesn't really end. As it closes, it is just a beginning.
>
> —Marguerite Duras

About a year before this book was published, a client colleague/friend surprised me with these touching words: "Your struggles have made you great. You're a fighter. You've made it this far. You're a survivor. Like a desert flower, you find the water you need in order to blossom. Your health crisis, as odd as this may sound, is like the water you needed to bloom."

Truth.

You, too, are blossoming. May this book be your sweet water. Cherry-pick the best tools from The Thriving Toolkit, get out a notebook, and start playing super sleuth. I hope you've already put some of the strategies into practice and are finding more healing, peace, and joy with every passing day.

The road goes ever, ever on. There will always be challenges and obstacles, but there is hope.

> Not all those who wander are lost.
> —J.R.R. Tolkien

Perhaps you were lost in the proverbial woods, but now you're wandering the path to healing, peace, and joy. My friend, that's progress. Bask in the glow of little victories.

This healing journey is your awakening to a new life. You have what you need—more wisdom than you realize—within you. It's time to call in your energy and step into your power.

Turning Our Healing Journey into a Ripple Of Good

Many ancient cultures believed each one of us has a bit of everyone within us. As we heal ourselves and bring peace to our minds, we bring healing and peace to our world—like ripples in a pond. In fact, just you being present is of great impact to the world. Never forget it.

We stand on the shoulders of those who came before us—our teachers and other wise ones. Personally, it has been a privilege to study the teachings of the many wise wo/men whose teachings echo through these pages.

We owe it to others to share our insights so they may climb upon our shoulders and be closer to the light. Share your insights with those who are struggling. Pass it on.

> The function of freedom is to free someone else.
> —Toni Morrison

If you need a guide to help you find the trail and not be sidelined when the path gets rocky—or you're ready to enlist a navigator—visit my website, SufferingtoThriving.com.

À votre santé! Here's to your health.

ACKNOWLEDGMENTS

Heartfelt gratitude to all my friends—too numerous to mention here—especially Carolyn Stevens and Heléne Diener and my husband, Ken Luber, for walking this healing journey with me, for listening, supporting, and encouraging me through good times and bad. Special thanks to Carolyn, whose suggestions, brainstorming, and inspiration helped me bring this book to life. Thanks to my publisher, Kary Oberbrunner, and the Igniting Souls Publishing Agency team for believing in this book, and my editors Erin Casey, Brad Fruhauff, Abigail Young, and my proofreader, Kristy Frazier. Big appreciation to my beta readers Dr. Kenneth and Sandy Browning, Carolyn Stevens, Kristy Frazier, and Ken Luber for their thoughtful feedback.

ABOUT THE AUTHOR

Kathy Harmon-Luber is an inspiring, compassionate, and empowering author and wellness guide. Her passion is helping people navigate the challenging terrain of the healing journey to heal themselves and the planet. With insight and enthusiasm, she opens people's eyes to the potential of becoming more physically, emotionally, and spiritually healthy by offering a toolkit of practical solutions. Her award-winning poetry, art, and photography have been featured nationally.

Visit SufferingtoThriving.com for ways to connect, her online gallery at KathyHarmonLuber.com, and shop https://fineartamerica.com/profiles/kathy-harmon-luber/shop.

NEXT STEPS ON YOUR HEALING JOURNEY

- ❖ Visit <u>SufferingtoThriving.com</u> for additional information, resources, and ways to connect on social media.

- ❖ Sign up for email newsletters that share helpful wellness information, new resources, and more.

- ❖ Experience one-on-one guidance with Kathy as your navigator: take a deeper dive into specific topics, reframe your health crisis, design a better future, or schedule a healing energy session.

- ❖ Create a healthier, more balanced workplace for your non-profit organization or business through Kathy's trainings and guidance.

- ❖ Order copies of this book for friends, family, colleagues, your doctor's office, hospital, hospice, and library.

SufferingtoThriving.com

ENDNOTES

1. Healing Journey Fellowship supporters: Carolyn Stevens and Joyce Grand, Heléne Diener, Bonnie Bedelia and Michael MacRae, Kathryn Carter and John Spring Covell, Lois Sheppard, Maia Bell, Robert B., Beth Tuttle, Scott Schroeder, Lynn and Joe Federline, Linda and Rolando Klein, Trudy Levy, Rochelle Devorkin, Marilyn and Ron Barlow, Minda Devorkin, Kirsten Stewart, Sandra Luber, Danielle Segura.
2. Martha Beck, *The Way of Integrity: Finding the Path to Your True Self* (The Open Field, 2021).
3. "Chronic Diseases in America," Centers for Disease Control and Prevention (Centers for Disease Control and Prevention, January 12, 2021), https://www.cdc.gov/chronicdisease/resources/infographic/chronic-diseases.htm.
4. "Toxic Chemicals," NRDC (Natural Resources Defense Council, August 27, 2021), https://www.nrdc.org/issues/toxic-chemicals.
5. William Braxton Irvine, *The Stoic Challenge: A Philosopher's Guide to Becoming Tougher, Calmer, and More Resilient* (New York, NY: W.W. Norton & Company, Inc., 2021).
6. Leonard Cohen, "Anthem," January–June 1992, track five on *The Future*, Columbia, 1992.
7. William Blake, *Songs of Innocence and of Experience, Showing the Two Contrary States of the Human Soul* (Basil Montagu Pickering, 1868).
8. Irvine, *The Stoic Challenge*.
9. Florence Scovel Shinn, *Your Word Is Your Wand* (Wilder, 2009).
10. Deepak Chopra, MD, *Quantum Healing: Exploring the Frontiers of Mind/Body Medicine* (Bantam Books, 2015).
11. Michael A. Singer, *The Untethered Soul* (New Harbinger, 2007).
12. A definition of *metanoia* is "to change our minds and lives as a result of spiritual conversations or learning."
13. Julie Tseng and Jordan Poppenk, "Brain Meta-State Transitions Demarcate Thoughts across Task Contexts Exposing the Mental Noise

of Trait Neuroticism," *Nature Communications* 11, no. 1 (2020), https://doi.org/10.1038/s41467-020-17255-9.
14. Jill Bolte Taylor, *My Stroke of Insight* (Penguin, 2009).
15. To be clear, if you do have symptoms of depression, you should put this book down and find help.
16. Singer, *Untethered Soul*.
17. Elizabeth Kübler-Ross, *On Death & Dying* (Scribner, 2014).
18. Salim Ismail. *Exponential Organizations: Why New Organizations are Ten Times Better, Faster, and Cheaper Than Yours (and what to Do about It)* (Diversion Books, 2014).
19. Scott Berinato, "That Discomfort You're Feeling Is Grief" (Harvard Business Review, March 23, 2020), https://hbr.org/2020/03/that-discomfort-youre-feeling-is-grief.
20. See, for example, *The Tibetan Book of Living & Dying* by Sogyal Rinpoche and www.dyingconsciously.org.
21. Carla E. Zelaya, James M. Dahlhamer, Jacqueline W. Lucas, Eric M. Connor, "Chronic Pain and High-impact Chronic Pain Among U.S. Adults, 2019," CDC National Center for Health Statistics, Data Brief No. 390, November 2020.
22. William C. Shiel, "Pain (Chronic and Acute)," MedicineNet (MedicineNet, June 13, 2018), https://www.medicinenet.com/pain_acute_and_chronic/views.htm.
23. "Loneliness and Social Isolation Linked to Serious Health Conditions," Centers for Disease Control and Prevention (Centers for Disease Control and Prevention, April 29, 2021), https://www.cdc.gov/aging/publications/features/lonely-older-adults.html.
24. There are many books on the subject, including those by Pete Egoscue and Dr. John Sarno.
25. Jon Kabat-Zinn is professor emeritus of medicine at University of Massachusetts Medical School and the founder of its Stress Reduction Clinic & Center for Mindfulness in Medicine, Health Care & Society. See his pain meditation CDs, books, YouTube lectures, and online resources.
26. Jon Kabat-Zinn, *Mindfulness Meditation for Pain Relief: Guided Practices for Reclaiming Your Body and Your Life* (Sounds True, 2009), compact disc; https://www.mindfulnesscds.com/.
27. Gabor Maté, *When the Body Says No: Understanding the Stress-Disease Connection* (Wiley, 2011).
28. Merle Shain, *Hearts that We Broke Long Ago* (Bantam, 1983).
29. Fenton Johnson, *At the Center of All Beauty: Solitude and the Creative Life* (Norton, 2020).
30. "Hygge English Definition and Meaning," Lexico Dictionaries | English (Lexico Dictionaries), https://www.lexico.com/en/definition/hygge.

31 Joseph Campbell, *The Hero with a Thousand Faces* (New World Library, 2008).
32 Robin Wall Kimmerer, *Braiding Sweetgrass: Indigenous Wisdom, Scientific Knowledge and the Teachings of Plants* (Milkweed Editions, 2013).
33 Explore the Native American medicine wheel, Frank MacEowen's Celtic spirit wheel, and the works of Alberto Villoldo and Sharon Blackie.
34 For exercises on tapping into intuition/synchronicity, read Robert Moss's *Sidewalk Oracles* (New World Library, 2015).
35 Michael J. Meade, *Awakening the Soul: A Deep Response to a Troubled World* (Greenfire, 2018).
36 Johann Wolfgang von Goethe, *Faust, First Part* (H. Böhlau, 1887).
37 Maté, *When the Body Says No*.
38 University of Konstanz, "Ten minutes of massage or rest will help your body fight stress" (ScienceDaily, September 18, 2020), www.sciencedaily.com/releases/2020/09/200918104305.htm.
39 Kary Oberbrunner, *Unhackable: Close the Gap between Dreaming and Doing* (Ethos Collective, 2020).
40 Ming Tai-Seale, Thomas G. McGuire, and Weimin Zhang, "Time Allocation in Primary Care Office Visits," *Health Services Research* 42, no. 5 (2007): pp. 1871-1894, https://doi.org/10.1111/j.1475-6773.2006.00689.x.
41 Frédéric Michas, "Time U.S. Physicians Spent with Each Patient 2018" (Statista, August 9, 2019), https://www.statista.com/statistics/250219/us-physicians-opinion-about-their-compensation/.
42 MayoClinic.com offers a free list of questions for your doctor, by condition, under "Preparing for Your Appointment."
43 In my situation, the likelihood of success was a hugely important question. When I inquired about surgery, I was told it would be a fourteen-hour surgery to rebuild my spine with very low odds of less pain or being more mobile, plus a risk of paralysis. Metrics informed our decision.
44 Syed Amin Tabish, "Complementary and Alternative Healthcare: Is it Evidence-based?," *International journal of health sciences* vol. 2,1 (2008): V-IX.
45 "Americans Spent $30.2 Billion out-of-Pocket on Complementary Health Approaches," National Center for Complementary and Integrative Health (U.S. Department of Health and Human Services), https://www.nccih.nih.gov/news/press-releases/americans-spent-302-billion-outofpocket-on-complementary-health-approaches.
46 Some medical societies and research organizations are American Cancer Society, American Heart Association, and Autoimmune Association.
47 Reliable sources of health information on the internet include MayoClinic.com, WebMD.com, Healthline.com, and TheMighty.com.

Also see websites for *JAMA* (the *Journal of the American Medical Association*), NAMI (National Alliance of Mental Health), IFM (the Institute for Functional Medicine), your regional/county mental health associations, etc.

48 Research prescription medications on Drugs.com and FDA.gov/Drugs.

49 For more information on an anti-inflammatory diet, see this article published by Harvard Health: https://www.health.harvard.edu/staying-healthy/quick-start-guide-to-an-antiinflammation-diet.

50 Autoimmune disease is the third leading cause of morbidity and mortality worldwide and now among the top ten killers of young American women. Autoimmune Association estimates that fifty million Americans suffer from one of eighty-eight autoimmune diseases—from type 1 diabetes to systemic lupus erythematosus—and some research puts the figure at one in five globally. At least forty more diseases are suspected to be immune-related. Most of them are devastating—frequently crippling, expensive to treat, and incurable. And they are increasing at an astonishing pace.
"Autoimmune Disease," National Stem Cell Foundation, https://nationalstemcellfoundation.org/glossary/autoimmune-disease/.

51 Steven Gundry, *The Plant Paradox: The Hidden Dangers in "Healthy" Foods That Cause Disease and Weight Gain* (Harper Wave, 2017).

52 Massachusetts General Hospital, "Reducing sugar in packaged foods can prevent disease in millions" (ScienceDaily), www.sciencedaily.com/releases/2021/08/210827082431.htm.

53 Huan Song et al., "Association of Stress-Related Disorders with Subsequent Autoimmune Disease," *JAMA* 319, no. 23 (2018): p. 2388, https://doi.org/10.1001/jama.2018.7028.

54 "That was the testimony given by the CEO of one of the largest pharmaceutical companies in the world. And interestingly enough, he was up for a 2.6 billion dollar bonus if he could produce enough profit." Adam Heller, "Pharma CEO: We're in the Business of Shareholder Profits. Not.." (ZPN), https://zeropainnow.com/pharma-ceo-were-in-the-business-of-shareholder-profits-not/.

55 Phillippa Lally et al., "How Are Habits Formed: Modelling Habit Formation in the Real World," *European Journal of Social Psychology* 40, no. 6 (2009): pp. 998-1009, https://doi.org/10.1002/ejsp.674.

56 Fenton Johnson, *At the Center of All Beauty: Solitude and the Creative Life* (Norton, 2020).

57 "Do Honeybees Sleep?" (British Beekeepers Association), https://www.bbka.org.uk/do-honeybees-sleep.

58 Jane Burnett, "Survey: 41% of Employees Feel 'Shamed' for Taking Vacation," Ladders (Ladders, April 11, 2018), https://www.theladders.

com/career-advice/survey-41-of-employees-feel-shamed-for-taking-vacation.
59. CellPressNews, "Researchers Identify a Gene Linked to Needing Less Sleep" (EurekAlert!), https://www.eurekalert.org/pub_releases/2019-08/cp-ria082119.php.
60. University of British Columbia, "You Need More Sleep to Find More Joy in Your Daily Life" (Regenerative Medical Group, March 29, 2021), http://news.regenerativemedgroup.com/you-need-more-sleep-to-find-more-joy-in-your-daily-life/.
61. Golden milk, a.k.a. moon milk, is a calming anti-inflammatory drink made with turmeric root, black pepper (to increase turmeric's bioavailability), nutmeg, cinnamon, and cardamom—adaptogens to reduce stress and induce sleep—in warm coconut or almond milk with honey or stevia syrup.
62. To optimize your sleep (or anything else), see Brian Johnson's www.Optimize.me.
63. *Wabi-sabi* is the ancient Japanese aesthetic philosophy of accepting the beauty of imperfection.
64. "Longanimity Definition & Meaning," Merriam-Webster (Merriam-Webster), https://www.merriam-webster.com/dictionary/longanimity.
65. John O'Donohue, *Beauty: The Invisible Embrace* (Harper Perennial, 2005).
66. Leon F. Seltzer, "You Only Get More of What You Resist—Why?" Psychology Today (Psychology Today, June 15, 2016), https://www.psychologytoday.com/us/blog/evolution-the-self/201606/you-only-get-more-what-you-resist-why.
67. Abby Rosenberg, Robert M Arnold, and Yael Schenker, "Holding Hope for Patients with Serious Illness," *JAMA* 326, no. 13 (May 2021): p. 1259, https://doi.org/10.1001/jama.2021.14802.
68. Bill Burnett and Dave Evans, *Designing Your Life: How to Build a Well-Lived, Joyful Life* (Knopf, 2016).
69. Joseph Campbell, *The Hero's Journey: Joseph Campbell on His Life and Work* (Joseph Campbell Foundation, 2020).
70. M.M.J. Van Hillegersberg and Martine Hofmans, "Consciously Training Our Gratitude is Good for Mental Health" (University of Twente, May 25, 2020), https://www.utwente.nl/en/news/2020/5/631059/consciously-training-our-sense-of-gratitude-is-good-for-mental-health
71. Malcolm Gladwell, *Outliers: The Story of Success* (Little, Brown and Company, 2008).
72. Search the internet for "gratitude research" and you'll find numerous scientific research findings about how gratitude changes our brains.
73. Pema Chödrön, *The Places that Scare You: A Guide to Fearlessness in Difficult Times* (Shambhala, 2002).

74 Elizabeth Howell, "How Fast Is Earth Moving?," Space.com (Space, September 1, 2021), https://www.space.com/33527-how-fast-is-earth-moving.html.
75 Summer Allen, "Eight Reasons Why Awe Makes Your Life Better," Greater Good Magazine (The Greater Good Science Center at the University of California, Berkeley, September 26, 2018), https://greatergood.berkeley.edu/article/item/eight_reasons_why_awe_makes_your_life_better.
76 Dana Sparks, "Mayo Mindfulness: The Health Benefit of Laughter," Mayo Clinic (Mayo Foundation for Medical Education and Research, July 11, 2018), https://newsnetwork.mayoclinic.org/discussion/mayo-mindfulness-the-health-benefit-of-laughter/.
77 Phillip Glenn and Elizabeth Holt, eds., *Studies of Laughter in Interaction* (Bloomsbury, 2013).
78 Ronald E. Riggio, "There's Magic in Your Smile" (Psychology Today, June 25, 2012), https://www.psychologytoday.com/us/blog/cutting-edge-leadership/201206/there-s-magic-in-your-smile.
79 Eckhart Tolle, *A New Earth: Awakening to Your Life's Purpose* (Penguin, 2005).
80 Wandering Travelographer, "Untranslatable Words – Qarrtsiluni" (Wandering Travelographer, September 17, 2018), https://wanderingtravelographer.com/2018/06/17/untranslatable-words-qarrtsiluni/.
81 "Robert Moss: Your Big Story Is Hunting You" (Excellence Reporter, May 4, 2016), https://excellencereporter.com/2016/05/04/robert-moss-your-big-story-is-hunting-you/.
82 Obviously, I derive some of these practices from traditions and philosophies that are not familiar to some Westerners. Don't worry about the specific terms and language; note, rather, the principle. You'll play sleuth and find what works for you.
83 Heather L. Stuckey and Jeremy Nobel, "The Connection between Art, Healing, and Public Health: A Review of Current Literature," *American Journal of Public Health* 100, no. 2 (2010): pp. 254-263, https://doi.org/10.2105/ajph.2008.156497.
84 Ronit Fallek, "The Power of the Creative Arts in Health and Healing," U.S. News (U.S. News & World Report L.P., September 29, 2015), https://health.usnews.com/health-news/patient-advice/articles/2015/09/29/the-power-of-the-creative-arts-in-health-and-healing.
85 "Keep Your Brain Young with Music" (Johns Hopkins Medicine), https://www.hopkinsmedicine.org/health/wellness-and-prevention/keep-your-brain-young-with-music.
86 Bridget Murray, "Writing to heal: By helping people manage and learn from negative experiences, writing strengthen their immune systems as

well as their minds," American Psychological Association 33:6 (June 2002).
87 Because I'm an over-achiever, I did manage to have a gallery show later that summer, though it required a lot of help from some very supportive friends and family.
88 Some courses I recommend are Flora Bowley's *Brave Intuitive Painting*, A Window Between Worlds's *Windows of Time* free workshop series (for healing from trauma), Chris Zydel's *Creative Juices Arts*, and Sheila Bender's *Writing it Real*.
89 R. Morgan Griffin, "10 Health Problems Related to Stress That You Can Fix," WebMD (WebMD, 2010), https://www.webmd.com/balance/stress-management/features/10-fixable-stress-related-health-problems.
90 XIV Dalai Lama, "Address of His Holiness the Dalai Lama at the Opening of the Conference on Seeking the True Meaning of Peace in San Jose, Costa Rica on June 26, 1989," *NewsTibet*, September–December 1993.
91 Shahram Heshmat, "5 Benefits of Boredom" (Psychology Today, April 4, 2020), https://www.psychologytoday.com/us/blog/science-choice/202004/5-benefits-boredom.
92 Frank MacEowen, *The Mist-Filled Path: Celtic Wisdom for Exiles, Wanderers, and Seekers* (New World Library, 2002).
93 Thich Nhat Hanh, "Rest in the River" (Lion's Roar, July 9, 2021), https://www.lionsroar.com/resting-in-the-river/.
94 Bees help pollinate the reported 84% of crops humans eat that are insect-pollinated. Amber Bragdon, "Bees Pollinate More than a Third of the World's Crops. Here's What Would Happen If They Went Extinct.," (Business Insider, August 2, 2021), https://www.businessinsider.com/what-would-happen-if-bees-went-extinct-2019-11.
95 Alexandra Sifferlin, "The Healing Power of Nature" (TIME, July 14, 2016), https://time.com/4405827/the-healing-power-of-nature/
96 For more information, see the Indigenous Wisdom library: https://indigenouswisdomsummit.com/library/8681; read books like Robin Kimmerer's *Braiding Sweetgrass*, and Sandra Ingerman's *Speaking with Nature: Awakening to the Deep Wisdom of the Earth*.
97 "Report on the Environment, Indoor Air Quality" (EPA), https://www.epa.gov/report-environment/indoor-air-quality
98 Kimmerer, *Braiding Sweetgrass*.
99 Dr. Qing Li, *Forest Bathing: How Trees Can Help You Find Health and Happiness* (Penguin Life, 2018).
100 Clinton Ober, *Earthing: The Most Important Health Discovery Ever!* (Basic Health Publications, 2014).
101 Wendell Berry, *The Peace of Wild Things and Other Poems* (Penguin Books, 2018).

102 Ocean Conservancy, Nature Conservancy, Natural Resources Defense Council, The Wilderness Society
103 Robert Moss, *Dancing with the Dream Bear* online workshop, The Shift Network.
104 C. G. Jung, *The Quotable Jung* (Princeton University Press, 2018).
105 Explore the work of Robert Moss, Dr. Bhaskar Banerji, Stephen Aizenstat, PhD., Alberto Villoldo, Sandra Ingerman, and Jane Burns.
106 Read tales by the Brothers Grimm and Hans Christian Andersen as well as the myths of your ancestral culture and folklore from other cultures. Explore Sharon Blackie's books and online courses.
107 Martin L. Rossman, "The Benefits of Imagery" (PsychCentral, May 17, 2017), https://psychcentral.com/lib/the-benefits-of-imagery#2.
108 According to one study, mindfulness based stress reduction (MBSR) as a mind-body therapy including body scan, sitting and walking meditation was effective intervention on reduction of pain severity and improvement of physical and mental quality of life. Maryam Didehdar Ardebil and Sudha Banth, "Effectiveness of Mindfulness Meditation on Pain and Quality of Life of Patients with Chronic Low Back Pain," International Journal of Yoga 8, no. 2 (2015): p. 128, https://doi.org/10.4103/0973-6131.158476.
109 Christopher Clarey, "Olympians Use Imagery as Mental Training," (*The New York Times*, February 22, 2014), https://www.nytimes.com/2014/02/23/sports/olympics/olympians-use-imagery-as-mental-training.html.
110 Patrick Cohn, "Sports Visualization: The Secret Weapon of Athletes" (Peak Performance Sports, October 13, 2020), https://www.peaksports.com/sports-psychology-blog/sports-visualization-athletes/.
111 Leonard Calabrese, "Beneficial Effects of Meditation on Inflammation" (The Institute for Functional Medicine, October 5, 2020), https://www.ifm.org/news-insights/lifestyle-effects-meditation-inflammation/.
112 Daisy Fancourt et al. "Effects of Group Drumming Interventions on Anxiety, Depression, Social Resilience & Inflammatory Immune Response among Mental Health Services Users." *Journal of Alternative Therapies in Health & Medicine* (March 14, 2016).
113 Isabel Pastor Guzman, "Tuning in to the Earth's Natural Rhythm" (Brain World Magazine, October 4, 2017), https://brainworldmagazine.com/tuning-in-to-the-earths-natural-rhythm/.
114 Masaru Emoto, *The Hidden Messages in Water* (Atria, 2005).
115 Water Science School, "The Water in You: Water and the Human Body" (U.S. Geological Survey, May 22, 2019), https://www.usgs.gov/special-topics/water-science-school/science/water-you-water-and-human-body.

116 Check out the works of Marla Leigh Goldstein and Christine Stevens as well as Layne Redmond's book *When the Drummers Were Women* (Three Rivers, 1997).
117 "Reiki" (Cleveland Clinic), https://my.clevelandclinic.org/departments/wellness/integrative/treatments-services/reiki.
118 John Beaulieu, *Human Tuning: Sound Healing with Tuning Forks* (BioSonic Enterprises, 2010).
119 Check out The Shift Network's online Sound Healing Summit: https://soundhealingglobalsummit.com/.
120 Check out classes by the Brothers Koren, Jeralyn Glass, and Eileen McKusick.

www.ingramcontent.com/pod-product-compliance
Lightning Source LLC
LaVergne TN
LVHW021801060526
838201LV00058B/3200